SURVIVAL
Symphony

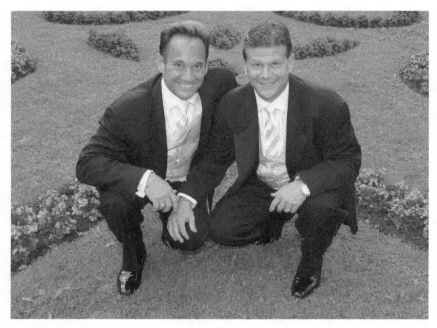

Louis and Scott Celebrating Scott's 50th Birthday at the Mirabell Palace Gardens, Old Town Salzburg, Austria, August 2013

SURVIVAL
Symphony
My Lung Cancer Journey

Louis V. Cesarini

ISBN: 978-1-736-5406-4-0

Design and production by Maureen Forys
Editing by Laurel Leigh and Sabine Sloley

Manufactured in the United States

Disclaimer: This book is based on notes and recollections of Louis V. Cesarini.
Some names, locations, and other identifying details have been changed or omit-
ted to protect the privacy of individuals.

 www.survivalsymphony.com

For my husband, Scott Simon.
Without his love, devotion and amazing
commitment, this book would not be possible.

Survival Symphony is also dedicated
to all stage 4 lung cancer patients.

Contents

Foreword

BY COREY J. LANGER, MD

I f attitude alone could defeat cancer, Louis Cesarini would have been disease-free within two weeks of his diagnosis. Since the onset of this unwanted and unanticipated journey in the world of oncology—eighteen months ago at the time of this writing—Louis has been indefatigable. He has approached his lung cancer diagnosis with tenacity and courage, and a unique, innate buoyancy of spirit I have seldom witnessed in my thirty-four years as an oncologist. Some patients have trouble coping with their cancer. This can affect caregivers and family by leaving them exhausted and deflated. Louis is quite the opposite. Louis radiates energy, even in the face of symptoms that would leave others defeated or depressed. The force field of energy and optimism Louis has generated elevates those around him. It revitalizes them. It makes everyone who cares for him feel part of the battle, invaluable allies in his fight, not just rote or perfunctory clinicians or practitioners. We need not tiptoe around the diagnosis or its implications. From day one, Louis has been fully engaged in this battle, and, I might add, incredibly engaging in his interactions with those who take care of him.

As Louis's medical oncologist since the summer of 2019, I have witnessed firsthand his spirit and strength. Cancer is a wily, formidable foe. It lays booby traps we often never expect; and the therapies we deploy to battle this disease, even while shrinking tumors, can cause side effects that will often sideline otherwise resolute, physically intact individuals. But Louis has remained unfazed. With his husband Scott by his side and the prayers and support of innumerable friends, coworkers and family, Louis has been able to wage every battle, making the transition from chemotherapy and immunotherapy to targeted therapy, dealing with life-threatening pulmonary compromise and spread to his brain and bones, always focusing on the activities that give meaning to his life, in particular, his love of the French horn. He has used his capacity to play this unique instrument as a gauge of his well-being. It's a personal metric. Every time he successfully completes a piece is another victory in this relentless battle. Hence, the title for this memoir.

While I've lapsed into clichéd military analogies to describe Louis's experience, he has appropriately and more specifically employed musical allusions to elucidate his life and his journey in the world of oncology. This *pacific* theme captures his life before the cancer diagnosis and aptly resonates with his experience since. Most pieces of music have well-defined movements; some end too quickly. I pray that Louis's *Survival Symphony* lasts indefinitely and that he be rewarded with the long-term quality survival he so richly deserves. I have promised him I will do everything I can to help make this possible.

Introduction

I remember being a little boy sitting on our sofa watching cartoons as my parents smoked one cigarette after the other in the kitchen, or when my dad would smoke nonstop in the car. The smoke made me so nauseous, but that's just the way it was back then. I love my parents dearly. They are gone now; neither one died of lung cancer. In the past, aside from early stage breast cancer, there was little patient awareness about lung cancer. Today, due to FDA approvals of new treatments, we are seeing an increase in lung cancer awareness. It is my hope that this book helps support this worthy cause. In my experience, many people react to a lung cancer patient similarly to how some people reacted to patients with AIDS: *they deserve it*. Certainly, hopefully, we can agree today that they don't deserve it and that it's a totally unfair assessment.

On the day I received my lung cancer diagnosis, at age fifty-nine, I was stunned with disbelief. I had done everything I was supposed to do. I exercised every day, ran a 5k once a week and ate healthy foods. I never smoked, and I have no family history of cancer. How could this be? I began connecting the dots of events that occurred in my life that may have exposed me to second-hand smoke or some sort of carcinogen that made me susceptible to cancer. Perhaps it was when I was age nineteen and in the U.S. Air Force, stationed at Grand Forks Air Force Base, North Dakota, guarding nuclear missile silos, or maybe back in 2012 when I lived in New Jersey, in an apartment above a garage that reeked of gasoline. I may never know the one or multiple causes, and knowing wouldn't change much. Once I knew what was wrong with me, I immediately went into survivor mode, drawing upon my oncology sales, training and marketing experience for the various available treatment solutions. That's what I want to tell you about in this book—how I chose to live, instead of accepting a death sentence.

I mention how music, specifically playing my French horn, has repeatedly helped me cope with tough times throughout my life. I was fourteen years old when my parents went through a painful divorce. It was playing my French horn and enjoying its beautiful sound that always made me feel good about myself. Over time, I grew away from my horn. This didn't bother me though, because in my heart I always knew that someday my French horn would be part of my life again. It was just sitting on a shelf waiting for me to pick it up. A few years ago, after a nearly twenty-five-year break from playing, I picked up my horn and re-taught myself to play. I had a great horn teacher in college, so I knew what to do. It was bumpy at first, but I knew that it would be like building blocks: little by little, that beautiful French horn sound would return to fill my heart and soul with abundant positive energy. Within months I was up and running, participating in the Curtis Institute of Music Adult Summerfest, performing on campus at Lenfest Hall. Little did I know that one year later I would be diagnosed with lung cancer. My French horn had returned in time to save me again.

§

Thank you for deciding to read *Survival Symphony*. It's nice to meet you in these pages. My full name is Louis Vincent Cesarini. I now refer to myself as Louis 2.0. I recently turned sixty years old, and if growing old is a precursor for being wiser, then I should be really smart by now. I have a wonderful husband, Scott. We've been together for twenty-seven years. I came out in the 1980s— what a crazy decade! Coming "out of the closet" during the AIDS epidemic was not fun. Unfortunately, I have encountered that same type of "looking down their nose" reaction from some people when they learn I have stage 4 lung cancer. If you share any of that experience, I recommend just smiling and feeling sad for those misinformed people.

Scott and I have shared a lifetime of dreams come true. I never believed I would get cancer, let alone lung cancer. At the time of my diagnosis, I was working for Merck & Co. as the PD-L1 Biomarker Promotional Manager. I know that's a fancy title that might mean nothing to you, but basically, I know a lot about how to predict whether or not a cancer drug will work. Almost two decades of oncology experience that encompasses oncology sales, sales training and marketing is what brought me to Merck. Upon being diagnosed myself, I knew I was part of a very small group of highly informed patients. I was well aware of what was to come and what to do. At Merck, I supported Keytruda, an immunology-oncology drug that has several FDA-approved tumor indications, including stage 4 lung cancer. Keytruda helps the body's own immune system fight the cancer. This drug could help save my life.

I believe there is no such thing as a coincidence. All the events of my life have led me to this moment of sharing my story. I believe the sole reason I am here today, living with lung cancer, is to share with you my particular skills and experiences that have provided me with the knowledge and belief that I can beat cancer. It's now my job and privilege to give other lung cancer patients hope. First of all, patients need to know how empowered they are. Treatment decisions affect our lives and our loved ones. We may be prone to rely on oncologists to make our decisions. Instead, these decisions should be made by the doctor and patient *together*. If you are a lung cancer patient, know that you have power and be ready to use it!

My life, as I knew it, will never be the same. I desperately want to get back to "normal," but as with the COVID-19 pandemic, I've found a new normal. I don't think of my cancer as something bad, but as an opportunity to make sense of my life events. In this book I share my day-to-day journey of survival, a bit like a diary. I peel back the layers of what I'm feeling along the way, connecting what's happening on any given day with what I've been through, always moving forward. Most importantly, I share solutions on what I did or am doing to maintain a happy, healthy, positive life.

That said, as my cancer journey began, I didn't realize what rough shape I was in until I completed the draft of this book and went back to reread what I had written. Some of my sentences and thoughts were incomplete. I had managed the barest of summaries on the days I was feeling bad. I guess we don't always realize how bad a situation is until we get to a better place and look back. Along with the support of my wonderful husband and friends, it has been writing and playing my French horn daily that continuously gets me through the worst days.

I've changed as a person during this unplanned journey. Scott and I have been through a lot. We continue to laugh like we always have, but some days are harder than others. My friends say that my positive attitude will help me win my battle with cancer. That always puts a big smile on my face. Don't get me wrong; I am scared. Although I'm getting better, and the cancer is going away, I don't know what lies ahead. The fear of the unknown isn't something that I think will ever go away. I try not to spend a lot of time in that space.

My experience and knowledge tell me that as a patient I have the power to determine my treatment with the goal of influencing my road to recovery. I've had no problem pushing back or challenging recommendations I deem reactionary or ironic. I've often been more positive than my community oncologist. Surrounding myself with positive people throughout my life, especially now, has been crucially important to my recovery. I encourage all cancer patients who have a community oncologist to also have an academic oncologist so no stones are left unturned regarding treatment options.

Some daily entries dig deep into my treatment experience. They're pretty intense. Each time I read these sections, I relive that day. However challenging these sections might be to read, for me or anyone else, they're an important part of the journey. These treatment sections tell my story as it actually happened so as to provide a real-world lung cancer journey. Fortunately, I've been able to move forward from these intense sections into some rewarding life experiences. I've shared a few of these as well!

§

Survival Symphony plays out in four parts: Discovery, Treatment, Courage and Believe. Each part parallels with the names of the four movements from Beethoven's 9th Symphony. Although other Beethoven symphonies could musically depict my journey, I chose the last one he wrote, no. 9 in D Minor, op. 125, as my inspiration for sharing my cancer journey with you. I've included suggested online recordings that refer you to the various classical music performances. I even include a few of my performances on the French horn!

I am humbled by all that I've learned about myself during the last two years. I couldn't have imagined that life's road would bring me to this point. I always knew that music would be an important part of my life but never realized it would play such an important role in my lung cancer survival, until now. I believe knowledge, proactive treatment and music are saving my life. Practicing my French horn has been nothing short of crucial to my survival. Playing my horn instills inspiration that makes me feel good every single day. I want to share my *Survival Symphony* and inspire others to have hope and live.

—LOUIS V. CESARINI
February 2021

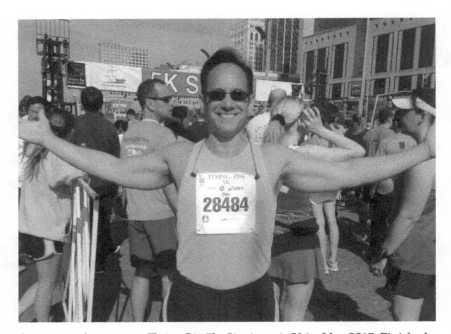

Getting ready to run at Flying Pig 5k, Cincinnati, Ohio, May 2015. Finished in 23:26 with an average of 7:34 minutes per mile; 6th out of 130 in men's 55–60 age group

Part I
Discovery

Movement 1
Allegro ma non troppo, un poco maestoso[1]

*In music, an instruction of "allegro ma non troppo"
means to play fast, but not overly so. Without the "ma,"
it means not so fast!—an interjection meaning slow down
or think before you act. The common meaning of "allegro"
in Italian is joyful. "Maestoso" means with majesty or in a dig-
nified way. Notice the unique way the symphony begins, growing gradually from absolute silence to a bold, dramatic sound.*

---

[1] *Music:* Beethoven: Symphony no. 9 in D Minor, op. 125 "Choral." The Mormon
Tabernacle Choir, Eugene Ormandy and the Philadelphia Orchestra (YouTube
video, 1:08:14). Posted by soy ink, August 24, 2017; accessed September 2020.
https://www.youtube.com/watch?v=eb_vUFxgtxM

I used to try to imagine how it would be toward the end of my life. What would it look like? Like some of us, I always imagined myself older, somewhere in my late seventies to mid-eighties. Dr. Langer told me that I compartmentalize. This seems to be a coping mechanism for me—putting my feelings toward someone, or some experience, in a metaphorical box, and putting that box on a shelf in the back of my mind to be forgotten, or stirred up when something reminds me it's there. I consider my doctor's comment a big compliment. I think of it as controlling the controllables. I might not be able to control what the cancer is or isn't doing, but I can ensure that everything else is positive and uplifting. I realized that I've been doing this much of my life, certainly from the time I came out as a gay man, until now.

I compare this first section of my cancer journey to the first movement of Beethoven's Symphony no. 9 in D Minor. The opening of this movement begins very softly. In musical terms it's called "pianissimo." It's followed by "tremolo": a wavering effect in a musical tone, produced either by rapid reiteration of a note, by repeated slight variation in the pitch of a note or by sounding two notes of slightly different pitches to produce prominent overtones. The opening steadily builds up until the first main theme of the movement powerfully reveals itself. This brilliantly depicts how I felt when I discovered I had lung cancer.

March 2019

Friday, March 29

Scott and I are heading to Hershey, Pennsylvania, to stay at the Hershey Hotel to attend a 2Cellos concert. We've waited over a year for this day. We missed their first U.S. concert tour, so this day means that much more to us. This is one of our bucket list items. Luka Šulić and Stjepan Hauser are virtuoso cello players. They are uber geniuses! Together they play beautiful music. We bought front-row VIP seats that included a meet and greet after the concert. Their performance is unbelievable! Scott and I feel like we are right there on stage. Our VIP meeting with them is a moment I will never forget. They are extremely friendly and genuine. Luka is very tall. When Scott goes to shake his hand, Luka opens his arms to hug him! They both have beautiful smiles. Hauser is funny as usual and is in true form with a wisecrack or two to share. Meeting 2Cellos is a dream come true of a lifetime.

Saturday, March 30

Scott and I run our weekly 5k in Hershey today. We always enjoy running when we travel. The various sceneries give us extra endorphins that add power to our run. Our running path today has gravel and steep hills. About two-thirds of the way through, I feel something pull in my back so we stop. Although we never stop in the middle of a run, I felt it best not to push myself. Scott and I are focused on meeting Eryn, the daughter of our good friends Cherie and Dean, for dinner tonight. Eryn just celebrated her nineteenth birthday a couple weeks ago. I met Dean at Merck while working on a project together. He was one of our oncology marketing directors at Merck. We've been friends ever since.

Sunday, March 31

I wake up this morning with severe back pain. I have never experienced this type of pain. I guess that the pull in my back I felt yesterday during my run has something to do with it. It reminds me of the car accident I had back in 2010, when I was rear-ended at a *Stop* sign and later diagnosed with a slipped disk. I underwent a series of three steroid shots over a six-month period. My back pain resolved, and life moved on.

APRIL

Tuesday, April 16

My back pain has persisted. Scott and I continue to run a 5k every Saturday. My back pain typically returns after each run and is gone a couple days later. Luckily, I have my annual physical scheduled today with my internal medicine doctor. (I will refer to him as Dr. Steve.) I tell Dr. Steve about my car accident in 2010 and my recent back pain. He prescribes Diclofenac Epolamine Topical Patch 1.3 percent, the same treatment I used to help relieve my back pain from my car accident.

MAY

Tuesday, May 7

My back pain continues despite the pain patch. I make a same-day appointment to see Dr. Steve. I tell him that my pain is now excruciating. I can barely stand up during the night to go to the bathroom. Dr. Steve is concerned and immediately schedules an MRI[2] for May 14. In the meantime, he prescribes a muscle relaxant, metaxalone (800 mg three times a day), along with 4 mg daily of Cadista, a brand of prednisone.

Dr. Steve's office submits the prior authorization[3] request for me to have an MRI. I have my health insurance through my husband's employer. Scott has excellent health insurance.

....

Monday, May 13

My MRI prior authorization is approved in time for my appointment tomorrow. Good thing, because the pain is excruciating. I've been sleeping on the family room sofa where it's easier to get to the bathroom. At one point, while Scott is helping me get up, I go to stand straight. I cannot straighten my back to stand up all the way. Pain shoots up through my spine, and we both hear a "crack"! We are so scared. I take an Aleve and walk around a bit, use the bathroom and return to lying down so as to relax. This helps, but I'm in a fog. It's hard to believe all of this is happening to me.

....

Tuesday, May 14

I completed my MRI this morning. Scott leaves on a business trip to Tampa, Florida, at 3:00 PM. He was supposed to leave on Sunday but postponed his trip until after my MRI. Twenty minutes after

---

[2.] Magnetic resonance imaging (MRI) is a medical imaging technique used in radiology to form pictures of the anatomy and the physiological processes of the body. MRI scanners use strong magnetic fields, magnetic field gradients, and radio waves to generate images of the organs in the body. MRI does not involve X-rays or the use of ionizing radiation, which distinguishes it from CT and PET scans. *Source: en.wikipedia.org*

[3.] The prior authorization process is used by some healthcare insurance companies in the United States to determine if they will cover (pay for) a prescribed procedure, service or medication. The process is intended to be used as a safety and cost-savings measure. *Source: www.spectrumhealth.org*

Scott heads out the door, I receive a call from my primary care physician's nurse, Jessica, requesting that I come in immediately to meet with Dr. Steve. I call Scott to let him know while he's on his way to the airport. We are both anxious. What can this be? Why the sense of urgency?

It feels like the longest drive of my life. Traffic is terrible. I'm so deep in thought that I miss my exit. Finally, I arrive at 4:35 PM. It is the end of the day for the doctors, so the waiting room is empty. Jessica comes out to greet me. She is always very kind and asks me where Scott is. I let her know that he's at the Philadelphia airport getting ready to leave on a business trip. She asks if I can FaceTime him. Now I know something isn't right.

Dr. Steve is an awesome doctor. He's very positive, always smiling, always energetic. I consider him my friend. Today he walks in with his head down. There's no eye contact, and he's not smiling. My thoughts race as he tells me that my discs are fine. Then he reveals what's on the imaging report: *The MRI confirms that three lesions on his spine are causing pain.* That "cracking" sound Scott and I heard yesterday was a bone fracturing at my T10. This area on my spine was weak due to the cancer lesions.

I know what that means. I not only have cancer, but I have stage 4 metastatic disease. How can this be? Me? The tears well up in my eyes and begin to roll down my cheeks as my mind continues to race about two hundred miles per hour. I want to go home, curl up in my bed, hide under the covers and cry.

Dr. Steve schedules a CT scan,[4] along with a specialized blood work request that includes tumor markers, for the next day. My poor husband is standing in the middle of the Philadelphia

---

[4.] A computerized tomography or CT scan combines a series of X-ray images taken from different angles around your body and uses computer processing to create cross-sectional images (slices) of the bones, blood vessels and soft tissues. CT scan images provide more detailed information than plain X-ray images. MRIs (magnetic resonance imaging) use radio waves instead of X-rays. CT scans and MRIs are both used to capture images within your body. *Source: mayoclinic.org*

airport in disbelief at what he just heard. I can't imagine what this is like for him. I just want to hold him. There's a lot of background noise in the airport as Scott struggles to listen to our conversation. We discuss and try to guess what cancer I have. The CT scan will confirm the type of cancer, but I think I already know: metastatic non-small cell lung cancer (mNSCLC). Me: a runner, in great shape, with no family history of cancer, and a French horn player. I don't know how I know the type of cancer. It's just the feeling I have.

I'm supposed to leave for downtown Philadelphia tomorrow to participate in this year's Curtis Institute of Music Summerfest. I'm to perform the second and third movements of the Beethoven Sextet in E-flat Major for two horns, op. 81b, with my French horn teacher, Jack. This recital will be a performance of a lifetime, and it's just five days away. The tears roll down my cheeks. How the hell am I going to do this now?

Dr. Steve knows about my horn background, and he knows just what to say. "Maybe this is the distraction you need," he tells me. What a wonderful doctor. He is also aware of my estranged relationship with my siblings and suggests that now might be a good time to reconcile with them. I smile, still crying. "No, I'm good. I have everything I need, but I'm sure my siblings would appreciate hearing you say that."

This is the most surreal experience of my life. At least now I know what's wrong with me. I dry my tears and go immediately into survival mode. My knowledge of oncology and lung cancer is powerful along with my positive attitude. After I came out in the 1980s, I was abandoned by my family and went on to make a wonderful life for myself. I survived those years without getting HIV/AIDS as so many did before we really knew what we were coping with. I think: All of this, and now you're going to throw cancer at me? I don't think so. Cancer picked the wrong person to mess with. It has met its match. Game on!

I tell Scott and Dr. Steve: "This is not how I'm going to die."

Wednesday, May 15

I fasted overnight to prepare for my CT scan. All went as scheduled. The results from today's scan will determine what type of cancer I have. Scott canceled his business trip and is back home with me now. I thought about what Dr. Steve said to me yesterday. He is right! Participating in Curtis Summerfest 2019 will be a good distraction. This is exactly what I'm going to do. Scott and I pack our bags to head to Philadelphia. For now, cancer will be in the rearview mirror. We book a junior suite for the weekend at the Sofitel hotel, which seems appropriate under the circumstances. Hey, if you've just learned that you have cancer, you might as well book a room at a luxury hotel, with high-thread-count bedsheets and room service to help ease your pain.

It's a bright, sunny day. Scott and I are in front of the Sofitel hotel in downtown Philadelphia when Dr. Steve calls with my CT scan results, two hours before Curtis Summerfest orchestra rehearsal begins. Dr. Steve tells me they found a 3 × 2 cm primary lesion on my lower ductal lung and another 8 mm lesion on my liver. My guess was close enough: I have metastatic lung cancer. Now we need to schedule a biopsy to determine what type of lung cancer I have: squamous or non-squamous. Dr. Steve works hard to schedule an oncologist appointment ASAP. Based on belonging to the Abington-Jefferson health system and having Dr. Steve as my primary care, internal medicine physician, I will be assigned to an Abington-Jefferson community oncologist. From here on I'll refer to them as Dr. CO. This is the normal process. I also know the value of having an academic oncologist as part of my medical team. Two of my friends from Merck, my previous manager, Kyle, and another coworker, Carolyn, jumped right in and reached out to one of the world's top thoracic oncologists at Penn Medicine (the University of Pennsylvania's Abramson Cancer Center at Perelman Center for Advanced Medicine) in downtown Philadelphia. I'm lucky to live so close. Some, if not most cancer patients, have to travel long distances to see their academic oncologist. My academic oncologist is Dr. Corey J. Langer, who graciously wrote the foreword to this book.

I head to the orchestra rehearsal. There are two Summerfest performance types you can sign up for: orchestra and chamber music. I signed up for both! I am among several other Summerfest participants performing in both segments. This year the orchestra is performing Beethoven's Symphony no. 4, first and second movements. There is one other French horn player attending, but I am assigned first horn for the Beethoven Symphony. The orchestra will have three nightly rehearsals leading up to our Saturday evening performance. After a second set of daily rehearsals for the chamber music portion, on Sunday afternoon Jack and I will perform the Beethoven Sextet for two horns. It's a lot of playing in a short amount of time.

§

Scott and I had canceled our original Sofitel reservation upon receiving the news of my diagnosis. There were several friends whom we didn't tell about my performance for this reason. We literally made the decision for me to attend Curtis Summerfest that day when we returned home from my CT scan. My pain was being managed and my will to participate overcame the decision to withdraw. So, here we are, and as we enter our hotel room, we appreciate its generous size. I can warm up on my horn in the sitting area before leaving for rehearsals. We always like staying at the Sofitel. The service is excellent, and the rooms are very clean. Chris, the hotel's restaurant manager, is great! We've come to know him during previous Sofitel stays. He will help Scott plan for an after-recital celebration at the restaurant on Sunday after Jack and I perform together.

I met Jack through his father, Dave, who also works at Merck. Dave is an associate director of oncology sales in the greater

Chicago area where he and his wife, Lynn (Jack's mom), live. I attended a Merck sales meeting back in March 2017. At a company reception on the last night of our meeting, there was a group of about six people talking. In the middle of the group, a gentleman was talking about his son who was a French horn major attending the Curtis Institute of Music in Philadelphia. The man talking was Jack's dad. My ears perked! I have a degree in French Horn Performance from George Mason University in Virginia. I studied with Edwin "Ted" C. Thayer during my time at George Mason. Ted was the principal horn with the National Symphony from 1978 until 2000. Jennifer "Jen" Montone, the principal horn of the Philadelphia Orchestra, also studied with Ted back when she was in high school. I was just a "few" years older than Jen when I studied with him. Jen is one of Jack's teachers at Curtis.

Curtis Institute of Music is among the best music schools in the world. Curtis students pay no tuition. They have donors who sponsor the students, so their tuition is paid in full. Curtis usually accepts only one French hornist per year, if that, and typically has over a hundred students auditioning for that one spot. Those who are fortunate enough to get into Curtis are considered prodigies. At twenty-three years old, Jack is no exception. However biased it may sound, he can go toe-to-toe with any professional horn player.

I listened to Dave talk about his son. He wondered if he'd done the right thing in supporting Jack's decision to major in French horn performance. Perhaps it would have been better for him to major in something like accounting. Given my own decision to pursue a career in biotech versus pursuing a professional music career, I couldn't resist interrupting Dave as I shared with the group that "his son will be fine no matter what." His French horn talent could be extrapolated into skills that would provide him a solid career. My life was living proof of this. I shared my degree credentials and background in music. The entire group roared with astonished laughter. Dave and I soon drifted away from the group and began a long discussion on his son's journey to become a professional French horn player. I really enjoyed meeting Dave. From that time forward, Dave, Lynn, and Jack would be bonded together with Scott and me, forever. This is part of how and why I returned to playing the French horn after a twenty-five-year break called "my career."

Scott and I were living in an apartment in Lansdale at the time, so it wasn't feasible for me to begin playing my French horn again. The apartment complex did not allow playing musical instruments. I also knew it would be a painful process for me and any listener to bear until that beautiful French horn sound returned. Regardless, I was committed to playing the horn again. Six months later, after we moved into our new home, I began playing my horn. It was good to have the French horn back in my life. The process was as I imagined it would be: painful. I had to re-teach myself how to play. I knew that I would need to be uber patient. It wouldn't happen overnight. I waited for Scott to take a week-long business trip so that I would be the only one to endure the painful process of achieving a good horn sound again. A month later, I began taking horn lessons with Jack at Curtis. Our goal became for me to participate in the Curtis Summerfest. This Summerfest program is for adults, like me, who are musicians and want to participate with other "like" musicians at a four-day master class-type program. By March 1, 2018, almost a year since I met Jack's dad, Dave, and after almost six months of playing my horn again, I submitted my audition video to the 2018 Curtis Summerfest.

Scott and I realize that I never had a new French Horn. I purchased a used Gebr. Alexander 103 nickel silver French horn during my first year of college at George Mason University. I was so poor back then it was all I could afford. If my playing improved, Scott and I agreed that I could look at buying a new Alexander. Well, it was January 2018, and my horn playing was sounding pretty good. I had practiced every day since October 2017, when I started to play again. It was paying off. Scott and I made the decision to purchase a brand-new Alexander. Here I was at fifty-seven years old, playing the French horn again after such a long hiatus and finally getting a new one. We reached out to a musical instrument distributor in St. Louis along with Reimund Pankratz, the sales director at Gebrüder Alexander, in Mainz, Germany, and placed our custom order for a new French horn. In order to select the best Alexander, Scott and I went to the factory in Mainz! They've been making French horns for more than two centuries, since 1782. It was a wonderful trip. Reimund and his staff were extremely helpful. They selected five pre-production Alexander 103s for me to try out. I selected number three! It's a real beauty. Great intonation and very pretty yellow brass with a screw-off flare. Having the ability to change the flare, or the bell, of a horn offers the player the opportunity to have different sounds depending on the metal alloy of the bell. Our visit to the factory and our stay in Mainz was memorable, one that will always be one of the happiest experiences of my life. My new French horn would arrive by the end of April that year, just in time for Curtis Summerfest 2018. It is a beautiful French horn! Its sound could be the envy of any professional French horn player.

I needed two contrasting pieces for my Summerfest 2018 application, so I decided to submit a video with me performing the second and third movements from Mozart's Horn Concerto no. 3, in E-flat Major, K. 447.[5]

I played the entire concerto as part of my junior recital in college. After all these years, here I was playing it again. Not a bad achievement for only four months of playing the horn again. I was very proud of this accomplishment. I looked at this period of starting over as an opportunity to be the best horn player

---

5. Mozart Horn Concerto no. 3 in E-flat Major, K 447, Romance (Larghetto) and Allegro. Louis Cesarini's 2018 Curtis Summerfest audition video (YouTube video, 9:07). Posted by Scott Simon, December 3, 2020. *https://www.youtube.com/watch?v=7rmLcf5u_Zw&feature=youtube*

I could be. I focused on intonation, quality of sound and, most importantly, breathing. My goal was to be a better horn player today than I was back when I graduated from college.

My first Curtis Summerfest in 2018 occurred in May. It was a wonderful experience. It was great being back playing my French horn with an orchestra and performing in a chamber group. I was assigned first horn in the orchestra. We played the first and second movements of Brahms's Serenade no. 1. The horn solo in the first movement is super cool. It was very exciting to play this piece! For the chamber group portion, Tania, a Curtis Clarinet major, and I, along with piano accompaniment, played Carl Reinecke's Trio for Piano, Clarinet and French Horn, op. 274. It is a challenging piece. One that truly pushed me forward with my horn playing.

Now, one year later, I enter Curtis's Lenfest music hall for the week's first orchestra rehearsal. I'm delighted that David, music director at the Mannes School of Music in New York City, is back as our conductor. David, a Curtis alumnus, majored in orchestral conducting. He has a positive attitude with a non-intimidating demeanor and great sense of humor that enables him to communicate well with the orchestra members. Corigliano's Elegy is another piece we'll be performing. I find my chair among the other orchestra members. I'm still trying to digest all that has happened over the past few days. I'm happy to be here though, and to be playing my French horn. This is where I need to be right now.

Corigliano Elegy for Orchestra is a contemporary piece. It's a bit atonal. As we rehearse I feel myself drifting, getting lost. My sound is crazy weird. I'm not sure what's going on. How can I be here? Where's Scott? I just want to hold him and cry and wish none of this was happening. I do my best and power through the Corigliano. My horn sound is horrible. Two-thirds of the way through the piece, just as I'm ready to literally get up and walk out, I notice that an Aleve tablet is jammed into my mouthpiece. I've been taking Aleve for my back pain and must have had a tablet in my pocket—where I always keep my horn mouthpiece. I start laughing.

....

Thursday, May 16

Despite getting eight hours of sleep, I wake up exhausted. The pain makes me pant like a dog. There's a Curtis faculty master class this morning at 9 AM, but I'm unable to make it to the rehearsal hall until 10 AM. Jack texts me, checking in to see where I am. I told him about my back problems a few lessons ago. This is all he knows at this point. I make it to the campus and meet him outside the door of Lenfest Hall. He offers to carry my horn. Although it's good to see him, I'm tired already and feel disconnected. Jack is a professional and a gentleman. He's always smiling and very positive. This helps me. He has an intellectual, mature approach to almost everything. I think of him as a forty-year-old man in a twenty-three-year-old's body. Jack is a great teacher. He articulates his direction well. He breaks things down so that anyone can understand. Jack is great at helping his students visualize what he is referring to. He's made me the horn player I've always dreamed of becoming. My breathing and control have improved dramatically. Jack is also a great listener. He understands how a student's mental and emotional states affect their playing.

As we enter the elevator to head up to our rehearsal room, he looks at me and asks if I am okay. The tears immediately run down my face. I tell him about my cancer. The elevator is still moving as his eyes widen with disbelief. He is the first person to know, other than Scott. Jack and I hug each other as I cry, both of us speechless for a few moments. When I can talk, I tell him that I don't know if I can perform our recital on Sunday. He assures me that I can. Jack says that I'm ready and that he'll be there with me; we will get through our recital together. This is just what I need to hear. I dry my tears as we head to meet our pianist, Michael, for our rehearsal. Michael is from the Washington, D.C. area. He's participated in

Curtis Summerfest before. He's a good pianist. The Beethoven Sextet, op. 81b is a challenging piece. Adding to this challenge is a piano part that is a condensed version of the string quartet; originally the Sextet was written for a string quartet that accompanied the two horns. There are a lot of notes! Michael does a great job. He is unaware of my situation. Jack and I never tell him. The three of us are there to play Beethoven, not to talk about cancer.

Dr. Steve calls me at the end of the day. He wants to get me in to see a community oncologist as soon as possible and confirms my appointment for Monday, May 20. Dr. CO is a newly certified oncologist. Dr. Steve tried to book me with a more experienced oncologist, but their calendars were filled and he didn't want me to wait.

I'm not expecting any more physician calls this week. Now I can devote all my energy to my horn playing so that I can play as well as possible. I need all my mental, emotional and physical energy to get me through my performances this week. I continue to take 800 mg of metaxalone three times a day along with Aleve and the Diclofenac Epolamine pain patch. This helps me, but any movements I make, including walking, are deliberate and careful. I will need to dig deep to gather all my energy. I've practiced so many hours. I've earned this. Game on!

Friday, May 17

My head is definitely more grounded today. The cloudiness is dissipating. I feel satisfied that our orchestra rehearsal went well last night. There is overall improvement in my playing today and my accuracy in the Corigliano piece is notable. It's unbelievable how much better a person can play the horn when there's not a pain pill jammed into the mouthpiece!

Scott tells me that there will be a big surprise today. I have a rehearsal break at noon. He meets me at Lenfest Hall and asks me to come out to the car. There, in the car, are our dear friends, husband and wife, Carolina (Caro) and Dan (Dano) from North Carolina. They came to see me perform in the orchestra concert tomorrow night. What a wonderful surprise! The timing couldn't be better. I find out later they planned this visit with Scott back in February, before my cancer diagnosis. We exchange hugs and kisses and happy tears. The sun is shining as we take a walk to Rittenhouse Square park. Once we arrive, I tell them the news of my cancer. They are visibly shaken and immediately commit to being there for Scott and me. This means the world to us. Caro and Dano have been wonderful friends since we met. They are family. I'm so glad they're here.

We head to Bud & Marilyn's for lunch. I order the chicken. I'm a bit uncomfortable on the bench seating in the restaurant. Without letting on, Caro asks Dano to go to the CVS around the corner to get something that can serve as a cushion. Unaware, I think he is going to the restroom. The next thing I know, Dano returns and hands me a CVS bag. Inside there's a watermelon beach towel that I can roll up to make a pillow to put behind my lower back to add comfort. That is so very thoughtful! I am much more comfortable now as I dig into the chicken, which is delicious. Eating well will help me maintain my weight. Body weight is a key performance indicator. Maintaining a good performance status is crucial at this time. The better a patient's weight, the better the chances that they can fight the effects of cancer and, most importantly, the side effects of treatment such as chemotherapy.

Before we leave the restaurant, Caro and Dano open up their calendars and pick a date when they can come back and visit us. We decide on a few days at the end of June. They book their plane tickets right there. We walk back to Lenfest Hall so that I can resume rehearsal. Caro and Dano head to their hotel. Scott joins them and then returns to meet me after chamber rehearsal finishes for the day. We head back to the Sofitel for a short nap so I can rest up for my evening orchestra rehearsal. Caro and Dano meet us at Lenfest Hall and sit in on our dress rehearsal for tomorrow's concert. The rehearsal goes well. Having Scott, Caro and Dano there is a big reason why. We all head back to the Sofitel for a glass of champagne and continue our visit.

I recognize that I'm in the solution. I am surrounded by a ton of love and support. I have the world's best husband, amazing friends and coworkers. With Dr. Langer, I have one of the best lung oncologists in the world. I am playing my French horn at one of the best music schools. I am exactly where I need to be. I have everything I need.

Saturday, May 18

Tonight is our Curtis Summerfest 2019 orchestral performance! I love Beethoven's Symphony no. 4![6] We're performing the first and second movements. Our performance goes well. It's surprising how fast a piece can come together with only a few rehearsals. This speaks to the playing ability of performers under David's leadership. Beethoven truly defines how I feel. That epically familiar first movement in his Symphony no. 5 in C minor, op. 67 is one of the other Beethoven symphonies that decidedly conveys the jolt I felt when Dr. Steve told me I had cancer. The movements that follow continue to speak to aspects of my journey. To me, the second movement is reflective, a pause. An opportunity to digest the news and develop a strategy for the journey that lies ahead.[7]

[6.] *Music:* Beethoven Symphony no. 4. Andrés Orozco-Estrada and the Frankfurt Radio Symphony (YouTube video: 36:07). Posted by hr-Sinfonieorchester, March 14, 2016; accessed November 2020. *https://www.youtube.com/watch?v=uGWklkORHJo*

[7.] *Music:* Beethoven Symphony no. 5 in C Minor, op. 67 and Beethoven Symphony no. 6 in F Major, op. 68. Yannick Nézet-Séguin and the Philadelphia Orchestra BeethovenNow Concert Series, March 2020 performance (YouTube video, 1:26:35). Minute 17:40 marks the beginning of the second movement in Beethoven's Symphony no. 5. Posted by the Philadelphia Orchestra, March 14, 2020; accessed September 2020. *https://www.youtube.com/watch?v=zKWYX5ohadQ*

Sunday, May 19

Today I will fulfill my dream of playing a virtuoso-level piece, side by side with Jack. I had a good night's sleep and wake up ready to give the performance of a lifetime. I've been rehearsing for so many months. I'm ready. Our performance time is 3 PM. I get to the hall early and spend some time warming up, breathing deeply and practicing mental relaxation, or what Jack and I like to call "horn yoga." I visualize playing impeccably, completely focused on how our performance will sound. Soon Jack and I are backstage, ready to perform. I close my eyes and imagine our performance as I finger the notes to the piece on my horn. We walk out. Many of our close friends are in the audience. I feel their uplifting energy as I enter Lenfest Hall. The only person I actually see is Scott, out of the corner of my eye. He is the person I am playing for first and foremost.

Jack and I begin the second movement. The second movement is slow and very melodic with the two horns answering each other throughout. Despite a few mistakes, I keep it together through to the end of the movement. The second horn opens the third and final movement in a horn call passage. I flub it up a bit but keep going. Despite my frustration, I maintain my focus. Just after the beginning horn call, around measure 27, a switch flips in my head. Who cares if I make a mistake? Maybe I'm at my most vulnerable, five days after being diagnosed with stage 4 lung cancer, but this is where I draw the line. I will not succumb to cancer or a few wrong notes. I think about how hard I've practiced. I know I can play this. And I do. From this point on, I'm sailing! Jack and I play the balance of the movement the best ever. I have tears in my eyes as we finish and stand to take our bows.

After the recital, Scott and I gather with our friends to celebrate at the Sofitel hotel. It's great seeing Lisa and her son Jake, Erica and Chris, Alisha and Will, Sarah and Ian, Steve, and Margaret and her friend, Ronnie Jean! I am especially happy that Jack is able to join us. Caro and Dano left in the morning. I can't wait to see them again. Jack is the only one at our soiree who knows my news. Scott and I decided not to tell our other friends just yet. Later we will reach out to each friend, one by one, and ask them to come by our home. This is how we'll tell them.

As far as my friends know, I've been suffering from severe back pain caused by a ruptured disc. Telling them the news one by one will make it challenging for me—I will have to relive the beginning of my journey so many times—but they deserve to know, in a time and place where they can digest my news appropriately and privately, versus having an emotional bomb dropped on them during our recital celebration. This was Scott's suggestion, and I agree with his plan. This day belongs to us, not cancer. So, Scott and I sit there, surreal as it is, knowing what we know, trying to enjoy ourselves despite this devastating news. I wish I would wake up to find that this diagnosis is a very bad dream. I'm sure this is how most patients feel about cancer.

Through it all, I am very proud of my performance. What I was able to achieve—the best performance of my life under the worst of circumstances—was like nothing I could ever have imagined.

Louis 2.0 was born today.[8]

[8.] A very special shout-out to my husband, who patiently recorded our chamber recital on his iPhone! *Music:* Beethoven Sextet in E-flat Major, op. 81b for two horns, Adagio and Rondo: Allegro. Michael Smith (piano), Jack McCammon (French horn 1), Louis Cesarini (French horn 2), Curtis Institute of Music Adult Summerfest 2019. YouTube video, 11:32. Posted by Scott Simon, August 12, 2020. *https://youtu.be/MtQTa3OWbt8*

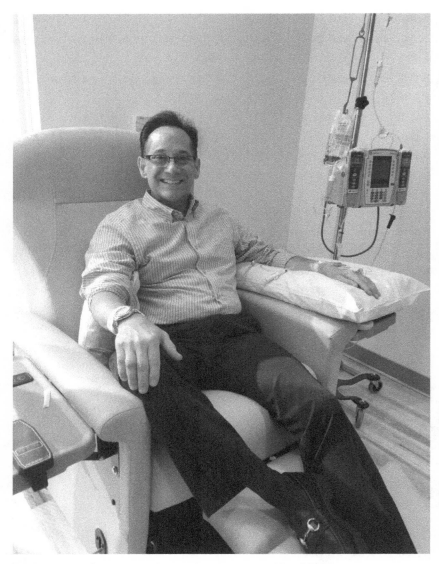

Receiving my first Keytruda Combo treatment, May 2019

Part II
Treatment

Movement 2
Scherzo: Molto vivace[9]

This movement is called "Scherzo," which in Italian means joking or playful. "Molto vivace" means very lively.

---

9. *Music:* Beethoven: Symphony no. 9 in D Minor, op. 125 "Choral." The Mormon Tabernacle Choir, Eugene Ormandy and the Philadelphia Orchestra (YouTube video, 1:08:14). Minute 15:16 marks the beginning of the second movement. Posted by soy ink, August 24, 2017; accessed September 2020. *https://www.youtube.com/watch?v=eb_vUFxgtxM*

W e all know treatment decisions are very important. Treatment decisions affect how we live with cancer. I've always believed that the right treatment should be given to the right patient. As I've said, it's a shared decision that the patient and their oncologist make together. Don't be afraid to ask questions; your doctor wants you to. It's not a one size fits all. It's important for a patient to understand all available treatments. Always be sure to consider side effects of a given drug. Treatments are a balance of risk versus benefit. If the risk outweighs the benefit, then why would we want it?

Back in 2003 when I began my oncology career, there were no drugs that showed statistical significance[10] for survival in metastatic non-small cell lung cancer patients. Today there are. Survival data is the holy grail for stage 4 lung cancer patients. Receiving an FDA indication for a drug based on statistical significance for overall survival in a clinical trial is rare. Be sure to check the FDA-approved package insert of the drug or drugs you are considering for clinical trials that have statistically significant survival information. Most treatments have side effects that may affect the duration a patient is able to take a drug. It is important to understand the trade-offs with side effects when considering one treatment over the other.

I've always been a glass-half-full, solutions-oriented type of person. I'm all for having a Plan A, B, C & D when it comes to handling challenges, so when stage 4 lung cancer arrived I put on my "solutions hat." I stay aware of the treatment options available to me. Each patient is different. I encourage every lung cancer patient

---

[10.] Statistical significance is a determination by an analyst that the results in the data are not explainable by chance alone. Statistical hypothesis testing is the method by which analysts make this determination. This test provides a p-value, which is the probability of observing results as extreme as those in the data, assuming the results are truly due to chance alone. A p-value of 5 percent or lower is often considered to be statistically significant. Source: https://www.investopedia.com/terms/s/statistical-significance.asp

to engage in a dialogue with their oncologist to better understand the "why" of available treatment choices. The treatments that I chose are *not* typical treatment choices for first- and second-line treatment of stage 4, non–small cell lung cancer. My first bronchoscopy histology results came back within twenty-four hours. They showed that I have adenocarcinoma non–small cell lung cancer. This is all the information I needed to begin treatment with Keytruda Combo.[11] We were still waiting for my ALK/EGFR and PD-L1 results. I didn't need PD-L1 results to start treatment with Keytruda Combo. Considering my back pain, I went with what we had. It took almost two weeks for my EGFR[12] results to come back. My ALK results came back negative the week before. I had no reason to believe that I was EGFR positive considering the small number of lung cancer patients who are.

The clock was ticking. I had cancer all over my body: in my lung, brain, liver, bones, lymph nodes, and I was experiencing severe back pain. Keytruda uses our immune system to fight the cancer based on approved FDA indications. My immune system needed help. It was compromised by the cancer. I stand by my

---

[11.] Please go to *www.keytruda.com/patientsite* for approved indications. Please note that Keytruda Combo is not indicated for first-line EGFR/ALK positive non-small cell lung cancer patients. Approved indications for all drugs mentioned, in addition to treatment protocols, can be found at *www.NCCN.org* (National Comprehensive Cancer Network). NCCN Guidelines can be found at this link: *https://www.nccn.org/professionals/physician_gls/default.aspx*. For more NCCN information on cancer drugs and treatment guidelines please register at this link: *https://www.nccn.org/professionals/physician_gls/PDF/nscl.pdf*

[12.] EGFR (also called epidermal growth factor receptor, ErbB1, and HER1) is a protein found on certain types of cells that binds to a substance called epidermal growth factor. The EGFR protein is involved in cell signaling pathways that control cell division and survival. Sometimes, mutations (changes) in the EGFR gene cause EGFR proteins to be made in higher than normal amounts on some types of cancer cells. This causes cancer cells to divide more rapidly. Drugs that block EGFR proteins are being used in the treatment of some types of cancer. EGFRs are a type of receptor tyrosine kinase. *Source: https://www.medicinenet.com/egfr/definition.htm*

decision to start with an immunology/chemotherapy drug combination first, based on how much tumor burden I had at the time. Today, I am having a remarkable response to the EGFR drug. I don't believe this would have happened as quickly had it not been for the immunology/chemotherapy drug combination I took first. Remember, there's no "one size fits all" solution, especially when you're the patient, and "guidelines" are just that, guidelines.

After finally receiving my EGFR results, they revealed that I am positive, with an Exon 19 mutation.[13] Approximately 15 percent of U.S. patients are EGFR positive. I am part of that 15 percent. What do I do now? I had already begun Keytruda Combo and I am having a positive response. I felt some pain relief within twenty-four hours of starting Keytruda Combo and 50 percent pain relief by the end of the first week. I discussed my treatment options with Dr. Langer. We decided that I would remain on Keytruda Combo. Feeling less back pain, coupled with the rapid response I was having were the main reasons. We made the decision to save the EGFR drug for second line in the event I had disease progression. Being EGFR positive isn't a bad thing. Now I have another option to treat my cancer if immunology/chemotherapy stops working for me.

I compare this second section of my book to the second movement of Beethoven's Symphony no. 9 in D Minor. The second movement is a scherzo and trio. A scherzo is a sprightly humorous movement in quick triple time. This scherzo resembles the opening theme of the first movement. You can feel the intensity building, taking off from where the first movement finished. This

---

[13.] An exon is a portion of a gene (sequence of DNA) that codes for the assembly of amino acids that are ultimately assembled into proteins. The EGFR gene, consisting of twenty-eight exons, contains the code for the construction of the EGFR protein. If even one of the exons is missing or mutated (exon 19 in my case), the EGFR protein is assembled incorrectly and can cause "EGFR positive" cancer. *Source:* National Human Genome Research Institute (NHGRI). *https://www.genome.gov/.* Please type the word exon into the search area.

intensity, for me, is characteristic of my treatment journey during the time I received immunology/chemotherapy. Certainly, we can agree there is nothing "joking or playful" about cancer treatment. Lung cancer treatment involving chemotherapy is no joke. The only thing that comes to my mind is that cancer is always jumping around once it's systemic, as with stage 4 lung cancer. It's a moving target, constantly looking for a place to settle. Based on my experience with the treatments I've received, it seems that when one side effect or cancer-related condition is under control, another one occurs.

An immunology drug coupled with the gold-standard chemotherapy combination is what I like to refer to as a one-two punch. This was the first time my cancer would have a wake-up call and stop spreading. We needed to hit it hard. I was thrilled to be in the solution. Every three weeks, I looked forward to each treatment knowing that each time I feel closer and closer to being cancer free. This made me very happy.

As I listen to the second movement of Beethoven's 9th Symphony, I imagine stepping back to think about what's going on and how I should respond. I'm not much for being reactionary. It's important for me to think things through. What is the challenge, and how can we overcome it? I look for all available clinical study information so that I can make informed decisions. I believe that clinical studies supporting a drug's particular indication are the best source of information as they pertain to a large patient population. This was my decision process for choosing the immunology/chemotherapy combination. To me, the beginning of my lung cancer treatment represented the first day of the rest of my life.

May 2019

Monday, May 20

My treatment journey begins today. I am extremely hopeful this journey will lead me to a full recovery—complete response (CR)[14]—and that I will be cancer free by this time next year. My appointment with the community oncologist assigned to me from the Abington-Jefferson health system is this morning at 9 AM. This is the health provider preferred by Scott's health insurance. I share my background in oncology with Dr. CO, including my current position as the biomarker promotions manager with Merck supporting Keytruda, a breakthrough immunology drug. I let Dr. CO know that I am consulting with Dr. Cory J. Langer, my academic oncologist at Penn Medicine. I don't want Dr. CO to feel threatened or uncomfortable, so I explain there will be a team of oncologists making treatment decisions on my behalf. It turns out that Dr. Langer was the attending physician for Dr. CO's fellowship. Dr. CO agrees that I should get a second and/or third opinion.

Dr. CO arranges an appointment with a pulmonologist. The pulmonologist will determine whether to do a biopsy or a fine-needle aspiration[15] so that we can determine which type of lung

---

[14.] A complete response (CR) to treatment is the term used for the absence of all detectable cancer after your treatment is complete. Complete response doesn't necessarily mean that you are cured, but it is the best result that can be reported. It means the cancerous tumor is now gone and there is no evidence of disease. *Source: https://www.cancer.gov/publications/dictionaries/cancer-terms/def/complete -response*. Please type complete response into the search area of this link.

[15.] Fine-needle aspiration (FNA) is a diagnostic procedure used to investigate lumps or masses. In this technique, a thin (23-25 gauge), hollow needle is inserted into the mass for sampling of cells that, after being stained, are examined under a microscope (biopsy). The sampling and biopsy considered together are called fine-needle aspiration biopsy (FNAB) or fine-needle aspiration cytology (FNAC). *Source: en.wikipedia.org*

cancer I have. My histology results will determine my treatment. Dr. CO informs me that a more comprehensive MRI needs to be done to cover my brain and upper spine. A PET scan[16] is also needed. I will complete these tests this week. My back pain continues. I need to begin treatment as soon as possible. With my heavy tumor burden, time is of the essence.

My community oncologist will not confirm that I have metastatic lung cancer until the bronchoscopy is completed and the histology is in. I tell Dr. CO that I know I have lung cancer, that it's adenocarcinoma and that I have a high PD-L1.[17] I have never been a smoker. I think back to a cough I had last August that wouldn't go away and wonder if that was the beginning of the cancer metastasizing. I know that about 85 percent of lung cancer is adenocarcinoma. I have no co-morbidities and am very healthy. The doctor doesn't understand how I would know my diagnosis. I just do.

Tuesday, May 21

I have my pulmonologist appointment this morning at 9 AM with Dr. Q, as I'll call them. It's at the same location as Dr. CO: the

---

[16.] A positron emission tomography (PET) scan is an imaging test that allows your doctor to check for diseases in your body. The scan uses a special dye containing radioactive tracers. These tracers are either swallowed, inhaled, or injected into a vein in your arm depending on what part of the body is being examined. Certain organs and tissues then absorb the tracer. The tracer will collect in areas of higher chemical activity, which is helpful because certain tissues of the body, and certain diseases, have a higher level of chemical activity. These areas of disease will show up as bright spots on the PET scan. *Source: https://www.healthline.com/health/pet-scan*

[17.] PD-L1 is a protein that allows some cells to escape an attack by the immune system. Extending from the cancer cell surface, PD-L1 interacts with a protein called PD-1 on important immune system cells called T cells. This coupling, known as an immune checkpoint, instructs the T cell to leave the tumor cell alone. Checkpoint inhibitor drugs prevent the PD-1/PD-L1 meeting from taking place. Without receiving the stop signal from the PD-L1 protein, the T cells can attack the tumor cells. *Source: https://www.cancer.gov/publications/dictionaries/cancer-terms/def/pd-l1*

Asplundh Cancer Center in Willow Grove. It's a new state-of-the-art cancer center. Dr. Q confirms that I will have a bronchoscopy and that it's scheduled for tomorrow at noon.

I receive a call from my community nurse navigator, who confirms that my MRI and PET scan are scheduled for May 28 or 29. I remind them of my goal to have all tests done this week so I can begin my first every-third-week cycle of Keytruda Combo the following week. The sooner my treatment begins, the sooner my back pain will go away.

An hour later, I receive a second call from my nurse navigator, confirming that they were able to schedule my second MRI for this afternoon at 4 pm. Additionally, my PET scan appointment has been moved up to this coming Friday. Now that all of these tests are scheduled, I can begin my first treatment cycle by the end of the month. Typically, this arduous process takes six to eight weeks to accomplish. It's hard for me to imagine any cancer patient waiting that long. I am in so much pain. I need to begin treatment now! I do all that I know I can do, based on my knowledge, to trim this process down to two weeks. I head to the lab for my second, more comprehensive MRI. It's done by 6:30 PM.

··

Wednesday, May 22

My bronchoscopy is completed by 2 PM. Dr. Q checks in with me during recovery to share that there is *no* sign of any cancer in my lung airways. He is quite surprised. I know the reason for this is because of my regular physical activity, running, and playing my French horn. I've kept my airways cancer free due to the consistent high volume of air traveling through my lungs.

It is a rough recovery. I am so tired and nauseous. I'm hungry, but the thought of eating makes me want to throw up. I'm almost delirious as I develop a fever that reaches 104°F. I know I should go to the hospital, but that thought makes me stress out. I am where

I want to be: home with Scott. He is so wonderful! He knows I need food, and since I have aches and pains—arthralgia and myalgia—and can barely move, he spoon-feeds me two small containers of apple sauce. I eat slowly so as to avoid throwing up. This helps a lot. My fever soon goes down and I begin to feel better. I am able to get some sleep. I wake up at 2 AM starving! I eat a ham and cheese sandwich—it's the best sandwich ever.

I feel like I have been to war and back.

....

Friday, May 24

I complete my PET Scan first thing this morning. Soon after, Dr. CO calls to tell me that my lung cancer is non-small cell adeno-carcinoma, based on the histology report. Adenocarcinoma non-small cell lung cancer is found in about 85 percent of patients. Squamous cell is a type of small cell lung cancer found in about 15 percent of patients and is considered to be more aggressive than non-small cell lung cancer. Now that my histology con-firms that I have non-small cell adenocarcinoma lung cancer, I know that I can begin treatment with Keytruda Combo. Dr. CO shares that my PD-L1 biomarker status isn't in yet and that it will determine whether treatment with Keytruda is advised. I let Dr. CO know that based on the clinical data from the Keynote-189 study (Keytruda Combo), treatment is for all comers, regardless of their PD-L1 status.

Based on this information, I don't have to wait for my PD-L1 biomarker test results. Dr. CO asks me whether I want to wait

[18.] EML4-ALK positive lung cancer is a primary malignant lung tumor whose cells contain a characteristic abnormal configuration of DNA wherein the echi-noderm microtubule-associated protein-like 4 (EML4) gene is fused to the ana-plastic lymphoma kinase (ALK) gene. This abnormal gene fusion leads to the production of a protein (EML4-ALK) that appears, in many cases, to promote and maintain the malignant behavior of the cancer cells. *Source: en.wikipedia.org* (Soda M, Choi YL, Enomoto M, et al., *Nature* v. 448, August 2007) until my ALK[18] and EGFR biomarkers results are confirmed before moving forward with my first cycle of Keytruda Combo. (These additional biomarkers will also help determine my treatment.) I am doubtful that I am positive for either biomarker. I think to myself that when I receive my ALK and EGFR results back, and if I am positive for either, I will discuss my treatment options at that time with Dr. CO and Dr. Langer. Tagrisso,[19] the newest EGFR drug, will be my Plan B treatment choice. It's always good to have options. Alimta and carboplatin, used together, were considered by many healthcare professionals as the gold standard for first-line stage 4 non-small cell lung cancer chemotherapy treatment prior to the approval of immunology drugs. Keytruda Combo consists of the immunology drug Keytruda used in combination with the chemotherapy agents Alimta and carboplatin. I think about all the cancer in my body today. I continue to believe that we need to hit the cancer hard with the introduction of my first anti-cancer treatment. After pausing for a moment with these thoughts, I tell Dr. CO: "I think you know the answer to that question."

I will begin my Keytruda Combo treatment by the end of this month.

....

Saturday–Monday, May 25–27

Scott and I enjoy a nice Memorial Day weekend. No alcohol for me. I've never been a big drinker, though Scott and I have accumulated a nice wine collection complete with wines from around the world. It's still hard for us to believe that I have lung cancer. All we

---

[19.] Please refer to the FDA approved package insert for Tagrisso at *www.tagrisso.com/*. Exon 19 mutation patients were the majority of patients in the Tagrisso registration study. The Flaura study provided the clinical information that supported the new-drug FDA indication for Tagrisso for first-line treatment of metastatic non-small cell lung cancer patients who are EGFR positive.

can do is move forward and focus on my treatment. We're in the solution now.

....

Tuesday, May 28

I meet with Dr. CO again to review my treatment schedule and complete blood work prior to my first cycle of Keytruda Combo. Dr. CO confirms that my first treatment cycle is scheduled for this Friday, May 31. Confirming a patient's ability to pay and having good blood counts are the tickets to receiving treatment. Blood counts need to be within the appropriate range prior to treatment to avoid severe side effects that might put a patient in the hospital. If your blood counts are too low or too high, your doctor may withhold treatment until your counts improve. Sadly, your treatment could be delayed if you're unable to pay for it.

Dr. CO reviews my PET scan results with me. The "lighted" areas identify where the cancer is. I have cancer on both sides of my clavicles, my sternum, all over my pelvis, throughout my spine and both femurs. Dr. CO mentions that additional positive lymph nodes were found. I ask: "How many total positive lymph nodes are there?" The silence is deafening. Finally, the doctor responds: "Too many to count." Scott and I are shocked. I say: "I guess we can agree there are greater than ten positive lymph nodes." Dr. CO has no reaction to my statement. Okay, I get it. The cancer is all over my body.

This is an example of how interactions can vary with community oncologists versus with an academic oncologist, i.e., Dr. Langer treats me like a colleague; Dr. CO treats me like a patient.

The nurse navigator reviews the side effects of the medication I will receive on Friday. I am handed a thick folder of printed-out package insert drug information for all the medications I will be receiving on each of my visits or "cycles" as they are referred to clinically.

Dr. CO confirms that my performance status is zero. This means I am a healthy patient going into my first cycle. This is the best place a patient can be given that side effects from receiving immunology/chemotherapy treatment could affect performance status.

After my appointment, as Scott and I are getting into our car, I see that he is visibly shaken with the news of my PET Scan. Holding back my own tears, I tell him, "Don't worry, that's the last time we're going to see all of that cancer."

Wednesday-Thursday, May 29-30

I get some much-needed rest. I continue using the pain patch and taking Aleve. I've been practicing my horn every day this week after a much-needed break following Summerfest. Performing that recital took everything I had.

Friday, May 31

Scott and I arrive at the Asplundh Cancer Center by 8 AM. I am anxious and excited to be receiving my first cycle of Keytruda Combo. I decided to return to work today and schedule several conference calls during my time in the chair receiving the IV medication. All goes well, except that the participants on the call can hear the buzzer that goes off whenever the IV bag is empty. I ignore the buzzer, as I am leading the call and prefer not to acknowledge the distraction. After the call, I decide not to schedule any more conference calls in the future while I'm in the chair receiving treatment.

I feel a cooling sensation in my veins as Keytruda is infused! I request the balance of information pending on my histology report: EGFR, ALK and PD-L1 status. The nurse navigator has no update and cannot offer a timeline for when I can have this important additional information. The answer I get is: "We have no way of controlling when we get this information. We send out for our labs." I reply that I am appalled to hear this. It's only my knowledge and experience that have enabled me to be treated sooner than patients typically would be. This is the last time I see my community nurse navigator. I'm certain that I made a lasting impression.

JUNE

....

Saturday, June 1

First cycle + 1 day, a.k.a. "organ day." I feel a sensation of heat on my skin just above my waist, on both sides where I believe lymph nodes are located. I fondly refer to this area as my love handles. Until today, I had been experiencing pain in these areas. I feel heat on my skin at other various areas of my body.

....

Sunday, June 2

First cycle + 2 days, a.k.a. "bone day." I feel soreness in the areas of my sternum, pelvis and hips. I stop taking the dexamethasone[20]— or as I sometimes refer to it, "dex"—as part of my post-treatment regimen. Typically, dex is taken the day before, day of and day after treatment to help mitigate side effects. My nadir[21] will begin to hit me the day after my last dex dose. As the dex wears off, fatigue usually sets in. I may develop a fever. If this fever reaches above 101°F, I'm supposed to call the doctor and go into the hospital. I

---

[20] Dexamethasone reduces inflammation and calms down an overactive immune system and is significantly more potent than prednisolone. Long-term use can adversely affect the way the immune system reacts. *Source: www.drugs.com*

[21] Nadir is a term that refers to the lowest point of anything. In medical terms, nadir could mean the lowest concentration of a drug in the body. With regard to chemotherapy specifically, it describes the point at which blood cell counts are at their lowest after a chemotherapy treatment. *Source: http://chemocare.com/ chemotherapy/what-is-chemotherapy/what-is-nadir.aspx*

begin to feel fatigued today. I also experience a mild fever, but it doesn't reach 101°F at bedtime, so I am okay, no doctor for me. I end up urinating no less than twenty times. It is a real pain getting up and down so many times during the night when I'm trying to sleep. Poor Scott. I can't imagine he is able to get much sleep, either. Thank goodness this is the only bothersome side effect I experience after my first cycle, so far.

....

Monday, June 3

First cycle + 3 days. I wake up feeling tired. As expected, fatigue has set in. Megan, the nurse navigator at Penn Medicine, calls to confirm my June 20 appointment with Dr. Langer. I am happy and excited to have this appointment confirmed. Dr. Langer sees patients on Thursdays, Megan tells me, and she will let me know if he has any cancellations the two Thursdays prior to my scheduled appointment. Megan confirms that my records—tests, blood work and histology—are coming in from Abington-Jefferson. I tell Megan that I still haven't received results from my histology regarding my EGFR and ALK. She is very surprised that I have begun treatment without this information. I tell her that I had back pain and a heavy tumor burden; I wasn't going to wait. I also share with Megan that I believe I have a greater than 50 percent PD-L1 and that I am ALK/EGFR negative. Nothing's confirmed yet, I'm still waiting, it's just my belief. Unfortunately, I experience a little nausea, enough to make me not want to eat. My appetite has been very good from the time I was diagnosed until now.

Later, I receive a voicemail message from my nurse navigator, who says that my PD-L1 is greater than 50 percent, and ALK is negative! This is exactly what I told my oncologist it would be. My EGFR status results are still pending, due to be in by the end of the week. Dr. CO will be calling me to discuss these results. I leave a message for Dr. Steve with an update, including that I have tearing in my left eye along with swelling and tenderness in my eyelid.

....

Tuesday, June 4

First cycle + 4 days. I continue to recover well from the first cycle of Keytruda Combo. My energy level is improving as my fatigue diminishes. I enjoy a good night's sleep. Last night I only had to urinate two times—yeah! My back pain has decreased from eight to four out of ten. This is fascinating given that it's only been four days since my first cycle. My hips and pelvis are not as sore today, though my right femur and sternum ache.

Despite this, I resume walking a mile a day. I always enjoy walking with Scott, especially on a sunny day! This is the extent of my physical activity since being diagnosed in May. No more running or exercising for me. My body's immune system needs all the energy I have to fight this cancer.

My primary care physician, Dr. Steve, returns my call from yesterday. He says my left eye irritation may be a side effect from my treatment. I confirm that the discomfort is moderate and that I have no loss of vision. My overall energy level is improving. My fatigue level is 50 percent better than yesterday, and my back pain maintains a four out of ten.

....

Wednesday, June 5

First cycle + 5 days. I continue to feel better. My back pain hasn't changed from yesterday. My energy level continues to improve as my fatigue continues to diminish. The antiemetic I've been taking continues to work. Antiemetics suppress nausea. I'm not throwing up or feeling like I have to. Despite some nausea, I continue to eat and sleep well, with the exception of a sensitive left eye and eyelid tenderness. All other potential side effects are nonexistent.

....

Thursday, June 6

First cycle + 6 days. My left eye feels better although it looks very bloodshot. I am able to open it more than yesterday. I will be calling Dr. Steve to let him know. Dr. Steve's receptionist makes an appointment with him for this coming Monday to examine my left eye. I continue to feel better and my reduced back pain is maintained. I have no soreness in my bones today.

Mid-morning, I receive a call from Dr. CO with a specific update on my histology results: my PD-L1 is greater than 50 percent and my ALK is negative, which I already know from the nurse navigator's call three days ago. The results also reveal that I am EGFR positive. I ask Dr. CO to pass this important information on to Dr. Langer. I look forward to my follow-up discussion with them.

This information may throw a monkey wrench in our treatment path. The NCCN guidelines state that all EGFR non–small cell lung cancer patients who test positive for EGFR should be given a tyrosine kinase inhibitor[22] or TKI for their first treatment choice. They are often referred to as EGFR-TKI drugs. Tagrisso's generic name is osimertinib. It is a type of EGFR-TKI drug. A TKI is a pill, versus immunology + chemotherapy. Despite this and although it's contrary to these guidelines—and I emphasize the word "guidelines"—since I have noticeable pain relief, I hold firm with my decision to continue with Keytruda Combo. My back pain is much more tolerable since I started the treatment. This is not an ideal situation. Histology results can take weeks; meanwhile, patients suffer while waiting. A patient's performance status can deteriorate dramatically during this time. There was

----

[22.] A tyrosine kinase inhibitor is a pharmaceutical drug that inhibits tyrosine kinases. Tyrosine kinases are enzymes responsible for the activation of many proteins by signal transduction cascades. The proteins are activated by adding a phosphate group to the protein (phosphorylation), a step that TKIs inhibit. TKIs are typically used as anticancer drugs. *Source: en.wikipedia.org*

no way I was going to wait. No patient should have to wait this long after being diagnosed with stage 4 lung cancer, especially if they have severe back pain and a heavy tumor burden. This needs to change. A patient deserves to have this information sooner so that informed treatment decisions can be made with their oncologists.

Around 8 PM, I receive a phone call from our good friend and my coworker, Dean (Eryn's father). I am surprised to hear from him during the evening; it's about 2 AM where they currently live in Switzerland. He says he hopes it is okay that he arranged to have food delivered from Laura's Pizzeria, a local Italian restaurant in Harleysville known to locals as Laura's Kitchen. Surprised, I immediately say "yes!" Three seconds later, there is a knock at our door. It is Dean, food in hand! This is just what I need, a surprise visit from a good friend! Dean is on his way back from the American Society of Clinical Oncology (ASCO) international oncology conference that takes place in Chicago every year around this time. We enjoy our dinner as we catch up. Scott and I discuss our plans to see him, Cherie and the kids for a summer trip in July to Switzerland. We can't wait.

I have tears in my eyes writing about Dean's surprise visit. The timing couldn't have been better. This is one of the nicest, most thoughtful things a friend has ever done for me.

....

Saturday, June 8

My fatigue remains the same, though I feel good. There is no change with my back pain. I continue to eat and sleep well. I am walking more each day. Scott and I are up to 2.5 miles now! Since my diagnosis, I have been walking a minimum of 1.5 miles a day. It's hard to believe that I used to run a 7.34-minute mile. This distance, 2.5 miles, will be my high water mark for now. Except for days when I reach my nadir and begin to feel fatigue, I am able to maintain my goal of walking at least 1.5 miles per day. The only exceptions were Sunday, Monday and Tuesday of this week when I was coming off the dexamethasone.

....

Sunday, June 9

This morning I have a low-grade fever of 99.9°F. I continue to rest and eat well. The weather is great! I wear a jacket, just to play it safe. Today Scott and I walk 1.2 miles!

....

Monday, June 10

I have my appointment with Dr. Steve this morning to take a look at my left eye. Upon examination, Dr. Steve determines that an ophthalmologist should examine my eye. He arranges an appointment for tomorrow.

I feel good in the morning and during my appointment with Dr. Steve, but soon after arriving home I develop a low-grade fever again and my fatigue increases. Today is the first day since starting treatment that I feel some discomfort in my lower back and hip area. I am unable to sleep in my bed due to my increased back pain. I decide to curl up with my favorite blanket and sleep sitting up in our master bedroom armchair. I am comfortable now and soon fall asleep.

....

Tuesday, June 11

The entire area of my left lower back is swollen and sensitive to touch. Scott and I are concerned considering how well I've been feeling. We hope that it is only temporary.

I have my ophthalmologist appointment this afternoon. My pain is enhanced by the uncomfortable waiting area chairs. I actually hear myself panting. Wow, this isn't good. I can't wait to get home. The ophthalmologist confirms that my left eye has an immune response similar to a trauma response. It is most likely due to a surge of medication related to my first cycle of Keytruda Combo. My treatment could cause this reaction. The ophthalmologist confirms that my eye has already begun healing and prescribes eye drops to further support the process.

By the time we get home at around 3:15 PM, my back pain subsides. I now have a low-grade fever of 100.1°F.

I take my pain and anti-nausea medication at 10 PM. Once again, I am unable to get comfortable sleeping in bed. This time, I move to our family room sofa. For the next couple hours, I experience excruciating pain. It is so bad that I cry out continuously in the throes of pain. I actually begin praying, and I don't pray. I say out loud the names of the people supporting Scott and me. I begin narrating our twenty-fifth anniversary vacation trip to Kauai last year so as to think of a positive distraction. My yelling increases in volume to match the pain I feel as I finally doze off and fall asleep. I dream about feeling a transparent shell of energy around me. Inside, I'm pain-free. Around 2 AM I actually wake up PAIN FREE! I climb in bed with Scott, who somehow has managed to sleep through my earlier audible sounds of pain. I sleep through the rest of the night.

Wednesday, June 12

What a night! I wake up feeling better. My back pain returns, but it is much more tolerable. I still have a low-grade fever of 99.9°F. Scott and I enjoy our daily walk despite this. I wear a jacket, and we end up walking 1.4 miles.

Thursday, June 13

My back pain continues to be tolerable. Good news, my low-grade fever is gone, and my overall energy level is better. I am eating well. Scott and I continue with our daily walk: 1.4 miles today.

Friday, June 14

Finally, today I have more energy and my back pain has decreased dramatically. No fever today! It's a beautiful sunny day! I have a good horn practice session. Scott and I walk over 1.7 miles!

Saturday, June 15

I continue to have more energy. I have less fatigue and less back pain. My appetite has increased, and I've been sleeping in our bed. Scott and I enjoy a nice walk on the Perkiomen Trail. We beat our previous high water mark of 2.5 miles with a 2.6 mile walk today! My horn rehearsals have evolved into daily physical therapy. What better way to know what's going on inside my body, specifically my lungs, than practicing my horn every day?

Beethoven continues to be the best composer to illustrate how I feel. On the car radio, Scott and I catch the last movement of Beethoven's 9th Symphony on our way home from running errands. Tears stream down my cheeks as we sit parked in our garage, listening to the triumphant ending. This symphony is incredible! I think back on the melodies of the second movement. They remind me of how I'm feeling today.[23] I wonder about the rest of my life. I don't know how much time I have left, but I do know that I have everything I need to survive: Scott, my wonderful husband and caretaker; a world-renowned academic oncologist; and the best friends and coworkers. I am hopeful that I have years left as I continue to be grateful for what I have today.

---

23. *Music:* Beethoven: Symphony no. 9 in D Minor, op. 125 "Choral." The Mormon Tabernacle Choir, Eugene Ormandy and the Philadelphia Orchestra (YouTube video, 1:08:14). Minute 15:14 marks the beginning of the second movement. Posted by soy ink, August 24, 2017; accessed September 2020. *https://www.youtube.com/watch?v=eb_vUFxgtxM*

Sunday, June 16

I have been using my eye drops every day since my appointment with the ophthalmologist. My left eye is much better with slightly blurred vision. The redness and swelling are gone. My energy level remains good. Now, my "love handles" are sensitive to touch. My skin is warm. I smile as I think back to when I felt this sensation, just after my first treatment. I believe this is Keytruda Combo working!

Monday, June 17

I wake up having enjoyed a good night's sleep. I immediately notice I had less discomfort during the night when I changed sleeping positions. This change is notable compared to any sleep I can remember since mid-March. My overall energy level has increased, and my back pain is the lowest since my journey began. Yay!

Tuesday, June 18

Any back pain I experience is centered on the lower right side extending upward toward my left latissimus. I occasionally feel throbbing in this area. Interestingly, I only experience discomfort in this area when I take a deep breath.

Wednesday, June 19

Today I am able take deep breaths without any discomfort. I feel more like how I felt while taking the pre-med dexamethasone dose prior to my first cycle, only now I'm not taking any dex. Feeling this good without any pill medication is great!

Thursday, June 20

The pain in my latissimus region has subsided. My appointment with Dr. Langer is at 4 PM today at Penn Medicine in downtown

Philadelphia. Meanwhile, Dr. CO's office calls to confirm the appointment for my second cycle of Keytruda Combo starting tomorrow.

Scott and I are anxious to meet Dr. Langer. We have a lot of questions. We first meet with Dr. Langer's fellow, Dr. Manz. I tell him about my cancer journey starting with that day in March when Scott and I took our 2Cellos concert trip to Hershey. Dr. Manz says he will share this information with Dr. Langer, so they can review and discuss prior to Dr. Langer's consult with us.

We finally meet Dr. Langer at 6 PM for about forty-five minutes. We enjoy our time with him. We review my journey and discuss treatment options. Later that evening at home, Scott comments how he didn't understand most of what we were talking about but could see that Dr. Langer treated me like another physician.

The assessment summary Dr. Langer gave me includes the following:

> *We recommend the following for your EGFR + metastatic lung cancer*
>
> - *Optimal first-line treatment for EGFR + metastatic lung cancer is osimertinib.*
> - *Immunology (pembrolizumab) and oral drugs like osimertinib carry a risk of pneumonitis (lung inflammation) that is much higher when the drugs are used in combination, or when the oral drug is given after the immunotherapy drug. The optimal treatment sequence for patients with EGFR mutations that received immunotherapy first is not known, although most prefer TKI followed by chemo alone or chemo + angiogenesis inhibitor (e.g. bevacizumab), with CPI reserved for 3rd line.*

- *You have already started treatment with carboplatin, pemetrexed and pembrolizumab (optimal first-line treatment for patients without EGFT mutations), you have a high PDL and appear to have a symptomatic response. We recommend continuing this regimen and obtaining repeat scan before cycle 3. This should be accompanied by a brain MRI, at some point.*

- *See radiation oncology for consideration of radiation to the brain metastases, though close observation is likely sufficient for now.*

- *Denosumab is a drug that has been demonstrated to reduce the risk of fracture and improve pain from bone metastases. Zometa (zoledronic acid) is likely equally efficacious. We recommend that you receive this drug locally (a Q 3-wk injection that can sometimes be spaced out over 3 months, after 4-6 cycles).*

During our appointment, Scott and I had discussed our July vacation plans to Europe. We're planners. Scott and I made travel arrangements for this trip in November of last year, six months prior to my diagnosis. Dr. Langer recommended reducing the duration of the trip so that it doesn't interrupt the timing of my third Keytruda Combo treatment cycle. Surprisingly, he didn't suggest canceling our trip. Instead, we talked about how important it is to continue to live our lives, as appropriate.

Based on our conversation with Dr. Langer, Scott and I decide to reduce the duration of our trip from sixteen to ten days, including travel time to Germany and returning from Switzerland. Unfortunately, this means we won't be able to go to Venice, Italy. Scott and I are sad over this news but quickly decide to spend my sixtieth birthday next year in Venice. Dr. Langer recommended a follow-up appointment in about a month. My next appointment is scheduled for August 1, at 2 PM. I'll have my next MRI and CT Scan from Abington-Jefferson for Dr. Langer to review by then.

....

Friday, June 21

Scott and I arrive at 9 AM for my second-cycle Keytruda Combo treatment appointment. We meet with Dr. CO prior to my treatment. This is the protocol for each appointment. First, we check in with insurance. Second, I have my blood drawn. Then we meet with Dr. CO before heading to the infusion center on the other side of the building. Scott asks Dr. CO if anyone from Abington-Jefferson will reach out to me post-treatment to check in and see how I am doing. Dr. CO says, "We don't do that. Patients need to call us if they have any questions or issues."

Scott and I look at each other in disbelief.

During my pre-treatment examination, I share with Dr. CO that I have a cramping feeling in my left calf, similar to a charley horse. Dr. CO's eyes widen during examining my calf. I most likely have deep vein thrombosis, more simply known as a DVT. Tumors churn out chemicals that may cause blood clots. A DVT occurs when a blood clot (thrombus) forms in one or more of the deep veins in the body, usually in the legs. DVT can cause leg pain or swelling, but also can occur with no symptoms.

An ultrasound is arranged to occur directly after my infusion this afternoon. My ultrasound appointment is at the Abington-Jefferson hospital. During my treatment, Dr. CO reviews my pain medication regimen and based on my liver enzyme levels from May asks me to reduce my daily dose of Tylenol. I am happy to do this. I certainly don't want to damage my liver as a result of any pain medication I'm taking.

Because of the trio of brain metastases that showed up on my May CT Scan, Dr. CO is concerned about bleeding in my brain that might be caused by using the blood thinners I now need in order to manage my DVT. I ask Dr. CO to call Dr. Langer to consult. The decision is made for me to take Lovenox.[24] Lovenox is a daily injection in the abdomen area. It can be stopped immediately if any bleeding of the brain occurs. My brain metastases are very small and most likely will not pose a threat. From this point on, I will have regular CT Scans and MRIs. PET Scans will only be ordered as needed.

If the ultrasound confirms I have DVT, one option is to be admitted to the hospital to begin Heparin and undergo twenty-four-hour observation before being released to initiate daily Lovenox injections at home. I do not want to do this. I believe that I will be fine with having the doctor prescribe Lovenox. Scott and I will pick it up on the way home from the hospital after my ultrasound scan. I share my preference with Dr. CO, who reluctantly agrees. After all, you can't force a patient to do something they do not want to do.

Scott and I are driving to the ultrasound appointment at Abington-Jefferson hospital when Dr. CO calls with the information that my blood work reflects elevated liver enzymes. I am asked whether I drink alcohol, which I resent as I previously shared that I had stopped drinking alcohol. I know better than to drink while taking pain medications. Noticing the offended tone in my voice, the doctor half apologizes, saying it is part of their protocol to ask. Dr. CO wonders what else could be affecting my liver enzymes. I share that I've been taking one Aleve every eight hours. As I say this, I realize that it should be one tablet every twelve hours. I'm not sure what I was thinking. I must have been so consumed with my pain that I had forgotten that the average daily dose is one Aleve every twelve hours. Dr. CO recommends that I reduce my

---

[24.] Lovenox (enoxaparin sodium) belongs to a class of drugs called anticoagulants (blood thinners) and is prescribed for prevention and treatment of blood clots (deep vein thrombosis or DVT) and chest pain. Lovenox may be used alone or with other medications. *Source: https://www.lovenox.com/.*

daily dose of Aleve to twice a day. I'm glad that we had this conversation and am happy to reduce my daily dose of Aleve. Sometimes we self-medicate without telling our doctors. This is a good example of how important it is to share all information with your oncologists so that they can make any necessary treatment decisions.

Opioids are discussed, but I immediately dismiss this option given the addiction rates. It turns out that my AST level is now 61 and ALT is 100. These clearly are elevated liver enzymes. Prior to our conversation, I was taking Tylenol 500 mgs once a day. Based on my elevated liver enzymes, I will be discontinuing the Tylenol. My ALK phosphatase[25] is now 403.

Here are my blood work results from back in May:

> *May 15—ALK phosphatase = 186 (range: 40-150); AST = 18 (range: 5-34); ALT = 14 (range: 0-55).*
>
> *May 28—Pre-first cycle blood work ALK phosphatase increased to 308 (range: 40-150); AST increased to 49 (range: 5-34); and ALT increased to 67 (range: 0-55).[26]*

[25.] ALK phosphatase, short for alkaline phosphatase, is a prognostic factor for monitoring the level of cancer in the bones. When abnormal bone tissue is being formed by cancer cells, levels of alkaline phosphatase increase. High levels of this enzyme could suggest that a patient has bone metastasis. *Source: www.rogelcancercenter.org*

[26.] Aspartate aminotransferase (AST): Also known as serum glutamic oxaloacetic transaminase (SGOT), AST is an enzyme that is normally present in liver and heart cells. AST is released into the blood when the liver or heart is damaged. ALT, which stands for alanine transaminase, is an enzyme found mostly in the liver. When liver cells are damaged, they release ALT into the bloodstream. An ALT test measures the amount of ALT in the blood. The alanine aminotransferase (ALT) test is typically used to detect liver injury. It is often ordered in conjunction with aspartate aminotransferase (AST) as part of a liver panel or comprehensive metabolic panel (CMP) to screen for and/or help diagnose liver disease. *Source: www.webmd.com*

I did not receive my blood work results from May until today. It's been over a month now; three weeks since beginning Keytruda Combo. I should have received them sooner. These results would have been helpful to me beforehand so that I could have understood the context of Dr. CO's phone call conversation. Moving forward, I'll be proactive and ask when my blood work results will be available to me at the time my blood is being drawn.

Since my ultrasound is positive for DVT, I begin my daily injections of Lovenox today.

Saturday, June 22

Second cycle + 1 day. I complete my last dexamethasone dose today based on the day-before, day-of and day-after doses required with each cycle. I feel exactly how I felt during the same time of my first cycle.

This time, due to lessons learned, I receive my pre-cycle blood work results from yesterday through the online patient portal. The report reflects what Dr. CO shared with me yesterday on the phone. Based on that conversation with Dr. CO, I think about my current pain medication and its effect on my liver. Moving forward, my goal is to avoid pain meds as much as possible so as to avoid any damage to my liver. I'll bite the bullet as much as possible. I am not sacrificing damage to my liver as a result of managing my pain.

Sunday, June 23

I begin to come down from my nadir just as I did after my first cycle. As expected, fatigue sets in as I discontinue the dexamethasone. Despite this, Scott and I walk 1.6 miles. I drink plenty of water and I feel better. It's fascinating how staying hydrated can make you feel better.

Monday, June 24

Today I am experiencing my worst fatigue day since my bronchoscopy on May 22. Here's a summary of how I feel today:

- My back pain continues to subside. It's been three days since I stopped taking pain meds.

- My pain is centered on my sternum. I can feel swollen lymph nodes near my right breast.

- My stools are softer. This is most likely due to initiating DVT Lovenox medication.

- I gave in today and took one Advil. Advil lasts for about four to eight hours versus Aleve, which covers eight to twelve hours. Aleve makes me constipated and affects my liver. Because of this, I choose to take one Advil at 6 AM with another at 2 PM due to my back pain. I decide this is the only pain med I will take post my June 21 second cycle.

- My left eye is back to 100 percent—yeah! My vision is clear. It is no longer blurry or red.

- I left two messages with Maureen, Dr. Langer's scheduler, to confirm my follow-up appointment.

Tuesday, June 25

Today I wake up feeling better. The pain in my sternum has lessened and there is no longer pain under my right breast. I stay off all pain meds. Those lymph nodes are no longer swollen.

Wednesday, June 26

I am more fatigued today than I was yesterday. I drink a lot of water, which somehow seems to alleviate the pain. Scott and I walk 1.5 miles today. My appetite remains good. I have been maintaining my weight since mid-May.

Thursday, June 27

I have more energy than I've had just prior to my second cycle. My pain is isolated to the back area around the left/right sides of my waist. I continue to drink a lot of water. My overall pain and fatigue are minimal. I continue with not taking any pain meds.

Friday, June 28

I continue to feel good today. I wonder if this is due to me discontinuing my pain meds. I believe there is a connection, interesting . . .

Saturday, June 29

Our dear friends Caro and Dano arrive this morning! This is the trip we planned back in May at Curtis Summerfest. Though I feel good today, we have no plans during their stay considering my condition. This removes any stress, and we can focus on visiting and catching up. We order pizza and salads from Laura's Kitchen. Since Dean's surprise visit, Laura's Kitchen has become one of our go-to places for takeout. As we enjoy our dinner, we watch one of Scott's and my favorite movies: *Priscilla, Queen of the Desert*. It's a funny movie about three drag queens based in Sydney who take a bus, "Priscilla," on a road trip to Alice Springs, Australia. It has some great one-liners, as one may expect in a movie about three drag queens! Caro and Dano love the movie! We laugh the whole time as we watch it! It feels good to laugh.

Sunday, June 30

Today we go to Perkiomen Park and walk over two miles! Caro and Dano are runners. Together they've completed over a dozen half and full marathons. What a fantastic accomplishment! Caro's also really into yoga. They love to travel and are big into celebrating life events like birthdays and anniversaries, just like Scott and me.

After our outing, I am fatigued and experiencing a little discomfort, most likely due to the increased physical activity. I sometimes tend to overdo it. Reducing my physical activity has been hard considering how much I exercised before my diagnosis.

July

Monday, July 1

I decide to discontinue taking Zofran, an antiemetic used to reduce nausea and vomiting caused by cancer chemotherapy treatment. I've been feeling nausea and have an upset stomach. I know, this makes no sense. Zofran is supposed to prevent nausea. This is the nature of drugs; sometimes they end up causing more of what they are intended to prevent. This along with realizing that Zofran is metabolized in the liver makes me decide that it's best for me to discontinue taking this drug, especially since it is having a reverse effect.

This morning, all of us snap into work mode. We jump on our various Monday morning conference calls prior to Caro and Dano leaving. Their flight is at 2:30 PM so they'll be leaving here at noon. I miss them already and feel sad. Scott and I are happy to have had more time with them during this visit. We share with Caro and Dano that we are planning a Celebration of Life, Love and Friendship party sometime in November to thank all of our friends for their support during my treatment. There is no delay in their decision; they're in! Dano's birthday is coming up. It's July 6, the same day as my mom's passing.

§

Mary Lou Cesarini died way too young. My mom had scarlet fever as a child, which created scar tissue in her heart. This later developed into cardiomyopathy, which caused her death in 1988 at age fifty. The real truth is that my father had an affair and left my mom with four children ranging from five to thirteen years old. This took a huge emotional, physical and mental toll on Mom that I feel put her in an early grave. As a child, I was not close to my mom. She was a quiet woman who never complained about anything. She didn't smile a lot. It was easy to personalize this into something you think you did wrong. I believed I was a good kid who always tried to do what was right and to be the best person I could be. I saw her pain. I felt she was carrying some heavy-duty life stuff, and somehow I knew even as a little boy that it had nothing to do with me. It wasn't my fault. Of course, this was easier to think than feel. Like any other child, I really wanted my mother to love me. It wasn't until I grew up and came out that I was able to really step back and look at our relationship objectively. I was more confident by then. I remember vividly our last conversation during a walk together back from the ACME market down the hill from where she lived. I was visiting from Alexandria, Virginia, where I was attending college at George Mason. I came back to Scranton to see her as much as possible. I remember that day as warm and sunny. We just started talking as we walked up the hill. My mom was not a talker, so this was a rare moment, the perfect time to tell her something very important. I told her that it was not "her fault" that I was gay. I knew she was blaming herself, and I wanted her to know this. She didn't understand what being gay was. I shared with her that the feeling of fireworks she felt when she kissed my dad as a young bride is the way I feel when I kiss a man. This helped her understand, but at the end of the day all she wanted was for me to be happy and not grow old alone.

She also shared something very personal and private. Something that once I heard it made everything that occurred during the course of our lives make sense. Her first born, my brother Vincent, died three months after he was born from pneumonia. He turned blue in my mom's arms. As a new mom, this devastated her. To this day she blamed herself for not dressing him warmer. All these years later, she continued to punish herself for being the cause of Vincent's death. I told her that it wasn't her fault. She did all she could as a mom. She needed to forgive herself. This was a defining moment for us, one that created a bond so strong that it continues to this day, all these years after her death. I love my mom; she will always be with me. She is helping me fight cancer every single day. Her love as my mother, her commitment to her children, are what keep me moving forward.

Dear Mom,

Please know that I feel you with me during this difficult time. I've felt you with me ever since you passed. I know you've steered me to be back in Pennsylvania working for Merck. You brought me to oncology in 2003. There is no such thing as a coincidence. You made sure that I'd understand cancer and that I could receive the best treatment. I feel your love and know that you're right here next to me. You were a wonderful mother. You loved your children. I love and miss you very much. I will hold the memory of you and what we shared that day on the hillside in my heart forever.

Love, your son,
Louis

....

Tuesday, July 2

I continue to feel better, though I wake up with a headache that is more of a nuisance than compelling. I chalk it up to the high humidity and summer heat. I refuse to take any aspirin; instead, I drink a lot of water, and my headache is gone by 10 AM. I call Dr. Langer's office and the scheduler, Maureen with Penn Medicine, confirms my Thursday, August 1, follow-up appointment with Dr. Langer.

....

Wednesday–Sunday, July 3-7

I feel good going into the July 4th holiday weekend. I continue to work full-time from home and am planning on going back into the office. Scott and I walk about two miles, as usual. I no longer need to take any anti-nausea or pain meds. I have another CT scan and MRI of my spine and brain on Friday and will have the results by Monday. My energy level remains good all weekend. Scott and I are very optimistic as to what the results of my scans will be. I continue to practice my French horn every day. Playing my horn continues to be a great source of physical therapy. I can feel that my breathing is improving!

....

Monday, July 8

This morning I receive a voicemail from Dr. CO regarding my brain MRI. I don't know how I missed that call. I listen, dumb-founded, as I struggle to understand the medical terms used in the message. I think that it translates to good news but I don't want to assume.

> There appears to be interval resolution of a number of previously identified small subtle scattered enhancing brain lesions. No appreciable new enhancing brain lesion is identified.

I immediately call the doctor to see what this means. It is the end of the day. Dr. CO has already left for the day. Fortunately, I am able to reach an on-call oncologist and confirm what these fancy words mean: There are no brain lesions. The cancer in my brain is gone!!!

....

Tuesday, July 9

I receive another call from Dr. CO with the results of my CT chest/abdominal/pelvis scan with contrast imaging. My primary lung tumor reflects a 30 percent reduction, and my lymph nodes reflect a 25–35 percent reduction in size. The lesions on my spine appear to have increased. Dr. CO is not concerned. CT Scan imaging can make it difficult to distinguish new bone from calcified bone. This is after only two treatment cycles. Needless to say, I am thrilled! These are *amazing* results based on my heavy tumor burden when I was diagnosed. I continue to experience little or no pain.

....

Wednesday, July 10

This is the third week of my second treatment cycle. I feel good. It seems like a pattern is being established. It mimics the third week of my first cycle.

I have been going into the office for work. It's great seeing all my friends and coworkers. I especially enjoy seeing the surprised looks on some of their faces. I get it, considering my diagnosis and the history of how stage 4 non-small cell lung cancer is perceived. I smile to myself with the belief that I am changing that perception. Stage 4 lung cancer is not a death sentence. It starts with me, here and now!

....

Thursday, July 11

I continue to feel good as I begin taking my day-before dose of dexamethasone to prepare for my third cycle of Keytruda Combo treatment tomorrow.

....

Friday, July 12

Scott and I wake up early for my 9 AM treatment appointment. My blood work results become available as I'm sitting in the treatment chair. They show an improvement—yeah! My AST is reduced to 28, from 61 last time, and my ALT is now 41, down from 100 last time. ALK phosphatase is at 463, slightly elevated from last time, 403. Dr. CO continues not to be concerned. Scott and I are very happy that my liver enzymes are back to normal. What a surprising organ the liver is with how it can repair itself.

Saturday, July 13

Today is my day-after dose of dexamethasone. I have some discomfort as I feel some activity going on inside my body. As with my first cycle treatment, I continue to experience the sensation of heat on my skin in the areas where I have cancer. My fatigue is minimal.

Sunday, July 14

I wake up at 3 AM with pain shooting down my left leg. The pain originates in my buttock area and runs down through my leg to my calf. Coincidently, this is where my DVT is. I wonder if there is any connection, since Dr. CO told me that my cancer caused DVT. I am unable to get comfortable or continue sleeping. I get out of bed and apply a Diclofenac Epolamine pain patch to my left buttock. This gives me enough relief so that I'm able to take a late-morning nap to catch up on my sleep.

§

As expected, I begin to come down from my nadir, having discontinued my dexamethasone day-after dose today. I feel fatigued. Despite this, and another hot day at 95°F, Scott and I visit my nephew, Anthony, and his wife, Fallon. They have a new baby boy, Milo Jack. He's about nine months old. Milo is their third child. Antonello and Stella are his sisters. The girls are close in age. They were born almost two years to the day apart with birthdays in June. Anthony is my oldest nephew. He is the only grandchild out of eight that my mom knew prior to her death. I have a picture that I took in 1987 of her holding Anthony on her lap. It ended up that this picture was taken a year before her death. It has a special spot on our bedroom dresser. Mom didn't smile often, but in this picture, she has a big smile.

Anthony is my older brother's son. Anthony's father is fourteen months older than me. I have two younger siblings, a sister and a brother. I am two years older than my sister and seven years older than my younger brother. As of this writing, none of my family members know about my lung cancer. Aside from my mom, dad and Anthony, my siblings made it clear years ago, when I came out as a gay man, that they did not accept this lifestyle. I was in my mid-twenties and really needed their support during those challenging years. They thought my sexuality was a "choice." Many years have passed without them in my life and today, I have everyone I need to help me fight cancer. Self-preservation helped me become the man I am now. I stand tall and proud of who I am and all I've been able to accomplish. Scott and I have created a life filled with dreams come true. Who could ask for anything more?

Scott and I enjoy our visit with Anthony and his family. He and Fallon always include Scott and me for the kids' birthdays and holiday celebrations. It is difficult for me not to share the news of my cancer with them. I want to tell them but decide against it. This visit is about meeting Milo Jack. I'll know when the time is right. I take our time together with Anthony and Fallon as an opportunity to share more about my work at Merck supporting Keytruda. I walk through the differences between Keytruda, an immunology drug that treats cancer, versus chemotherapy. I haven't shared this kind of in-depth information about my work in past visits. Scott and I thought it would be a good foundation for when the day comes that they do find out. We return home. Exhausted, I take another nap and wake up feeling rested. I have a good horn rehearsal as I reflect on our visit.

....

Monday–Tuesday, July 15–16

Both days are typical of the days that follow my cycle treatment. I experience fatigue and some discomfort and pain in my hips and pelvis area. I continue to go into the office and work full-time.

Wednesday, July 17

I wake up feeling a little detached and fatigued. The discomfort in my hip and pelvis area continues. My overall pain, however, is relatively nonexistent. I have a dental appointment this morning and plan on going into the office for the balance of my day.

The weather continues to be hot outside with the temperature at 95°F. The air quality is poor. I wonder if this is impacting my fatigue and discomfort.

Thursday, July 18

It's been raining most of the day. After work, I practice excerpts from Beethoven Symphony no. 6. This is my favorite symphony. I love the horn solo at the beginning of the fifth movement. It's the sun coming out after the "storm." Today I play it better than I ever have. Tears well up in my eyes. I imagine this is how it might sound ascending to heaven.[27]

Friday, July 19

I continue to feel better. Scott and I are leaving for our Germany and Switzerland trip tomorrow. I have no fatigue or discomfort; as a result, I have a very productive workday. I enjoy one last horn practice this evening before leaving. I won't be taking my horn on our trip. I'll enjoy our time together away and look forward resuming my horn practice when we return home.

[27.] *Music:* Beethoven Symphony no. 5 in C Minor, op. 67 and Beethoven Symphony no. 6 in F Major, op. 68. Yannick Nézet-Séguin and the Philadelphia Orchestra BeethovenNow Concert Series, March 2020 performance (YouTube video, 1:26:35). Minute 1:16:57 marks the beginning of the fifth movement of Beethoven's Symphony no. 6 in F Major, op. 68 "Pastoral." Posted by the Philadelphia Orchestra, March 14, 2020; accessed September 2020. *https://www.youtube.com/watch?v=zKWYX5ohadQ.*

Saturday, July 20

Scott and I wake up early and finish packing for our trip. To avoid any back pain, we will be packing as light as possible so as not to have Scott carry all the bags. We arrive at Newark Airport in plenty of time to catch our flight to Frankfurt. It's hard to believe with all we've been through since then that we're still going on this trip.

Today, I really feel great! The timing of this trip couldn't have been better. We're not sure if the excitement from our trip has anything to do with how I feel, but who cares, we're going to enjoy our time away as much as possible. I can honestly say that for the first time since my diagnosis, I feel cancer free! Last night I remember dreaming and saying these words: "The cancer is going away. I'm beating this. I will be cancer free."

After so many years in oncology discussing lung cancer patient types, it's surreal to actually be "that" patient. Exercising regularly throughout most of my life, I've developed the ability to be in tune with my body. I can feel what's going on inside. I listen to my body, especially now. I am very conscious about getting plenty of rest, drinking plenty of water and eating regularly. I can feel that my metabolism has increased. This is probably due to the extra-hard work my immune system is doing to fight the cancer.

All patients need to realize that they have a seat at the table. My knowledge and experience in oncology, particularly with lung cancer, is steering my treatment course appropriately as an informed patient. I desperately want to help others who may not have this knowledge. This continues to be the primary goal of this book. So, the lesson for today is: Do not underestimate the power of a patient!

Sunday, July 21

Our red-eye flight to Germany goes well. Scott and I are able to get a little rest on the flight. We land in Frankfurt and take a train directly from the airport to Mainz. It's about a forty-minute train ride. This is our second trip to the Gebr. Alexander factory in Mainz. My old college French horn is a vintage Alexander 103, their most popular type, circa 1940s to early 1950s. It's at least seventy years old. I shipped it to Gebr. Alexander back in March, prior to my diagnosis. Now Scott and I are here to see my newly refurbished college Alexander! Although Scott and I have formed a good relationship with Reimund and Casper at Alexander, they do not know about my lung cancer. We will keep it that way for now. Unfortunately, our shortened time here coincides with Reimund's personal holiday. He will be away during our visit. Casper will be meeting us in his absence. He made us feel most welcome on our last visit when I picked out my new horn. We'll miss seeing Reimund during this visit.

We arrive at the Hyatt Regency; this is where we stayed when we were here back in February of last year. We enjoyed that first trip so much that we said we would have to return in the summer when it's nice and warm. The Mainz Hyatt Regency is located right on the Rhine River, so a nice breeze is always present. We definitely get what we were looking for regarding warmer weather. In fact, most of Europe is experiencing a heatwave. It's hot; about 95°F. We settle in our room and take a nap to make up for the sleep we didn't get on the red-eye. Since our room overlooks the Rhine, the sun is shining directly in our room. We crank up the air-conditioning to keep the room cool.

I continue to feel good but am tired. Scott and I both feel rested after our nap. We venture out for a walk around downtown Mainz. It's a very charming town. The square around the cathedral is quaint, classic European. We enjoy a nice dinner at the hotel restaurant, Bell Pepper. The food is great, and the service is excellent. We order an Aperol Spritz for our pre-dinner cocktail. This is the first drink I've had since my diagnosis. Cheers! Based on the recommendation from our server, we order a nice German white to accompany our fish entree. The fish is especially good! Scott and I very much enjoy our dinner. It's nice to be back.

Monday, July 22

Scott and I wake up early and enjoy a full breakfast. Then we're off to Gebr. Alexander with great anticipation. My "used" Alexander should look good as new and continue to sound great! Prior to the refurbishing, my college horn was tarnished throughout. It definitely showed the wear from playing all these years. There were some minor dents. The nickel-silver lacquered finish is worn. The lacquer and dents are being removed as part of the refurbishment. The Lawson lead pipe, the first section from the mouthpiece to the horn, is being replaced with an Alexander lead pipe. The rotors or valves are being redone as well.

Scott and I enjoy our time at Gebr. Alexander. Casper is very helpful, very professional and personable. I have tears in my eyes as he presents my refurbished college Alexander. After so many years, it looks brand new and sounds great! Scott and I are thrilled. I'm so glad we are here together to enjoy this experience.

Tuesday, July 23

It's another beautiful day here in Mainz! Scott and I spend the day walking around town. There is an outdoor open-air market in the town square near the cathedral. The smells of garlic, fresh raspberries, strawberries and fragrant flowers fill the air on a sunny, breezy day. We enjoy a nice dinner at a local Italian restaurant. Only outside seating is available. They're not big on indoor air-conditioned seating here. Scott and I don't mind sitting outside. What we do mind is that everyone, and I mean everyone, is smoking. Cigarette smoke has always bothered us, and since my diagnosis, it bothers us more. It's very humid outside and there's no breeze. I almost choke from the cigarette smoke. We hurry and finish our dinner.

Wednesday, July 24

Today we leave for Stuttgart, where we will see Scott's cousin, Ira, and his coworker, Gus. Gus and his wife, Maggie, and their newborn daughter, Martina (Tina), recently moved from Bogota, Colombia, to Stuttgart. Scott met Gus through his work, supporting a project they worked on together.

We stay at Le Meridien hotel in Stuttgart. It's a very nice hotel but for some reason the hotel restaurant is not connected to the hotel. The only way to get to it is to go outside the hotel and walk up about one hundred steps! There is a bar-restaurant off of the lobby along with a separate area for breakfast and lunch, but nothing more in the hotel where you could have dinner. By this time in our trip, I'm feeling some fatigue. It was bound to happen given that I haven't been this active in months. I do okay despite this, but the steps and heat aren't making it easy. Scott is great the whole time. He is always very patient, caring, and right there to help me. I love him so much.

Thursday, July 25

After a good night's sleep, Scott and I enjoy breakfast and prepare for our visit with Ira, Gus, Maggie, and Tina. We venture out to a local liquor store to buy a couple bottles of Veuve Clicquot to celebrate our reunion. Veuve Clicquot champagne is one of our favorites. The distance isn't too far, but it's all uphill, which makes it challenging for me. I am tired but power through and enjoy our walk. The liquor store does not take credit cards, so Scott and I have to walk to a bank for an ATM. This isn't too far from the liquor store, but we have to walk down a big hill and, yes, walk right back up it to return to the liquor store. All is good though. The liquor store owner is very nice. Scott and I are glad we were able to find one so that we can have a good champagne to celebrate with our friends and family. Ira is the first to meet us. We meet around 1 PM in the hotel lobby so as to have our celebration in the bar restaurant. It is quiet there, so we have plenty of room and uninterrupted time together.

Ira is a retired violist. While studying at the Cincinnati Conservatory of music, he left the States to join a German orchestra. We last saw Ira during our first visit to Mainz. He took the train up to see us. It's about a three-hour train ride to Mainz from Stuttgart. Soon after we meet Ira, Gus, Maggie and Tina arrive. They live outside of Stuttgart about a forty-minute train ride away. Despite the heat, distance and having a one-year-old, they come into town to see us. They present us with a beautiful authentic German stein. Scott and I found a really cute stuffed tiger at a children's store in Mainz. They choose the name "Slou" for the tiger, after Scott and Louis! We are honored.

After our lunch, Scott and I grab another nap before reconvening with Ira and his girlfriend, Ines. They've been together for about ten years. We take a taxi to the restaurant Ira chose. It isn't too far from our hotel. We enjoy our dinner. Ira and Ines are big walkers. I'm a little worse for wear at this point, and Scott and I reluctantly agree to walk with them back to our hotel. It is another hot, humid evening, and I walk very slowly. Ira and Ines are very patient and keep the pace where I am comfortable. After dinner we enjoy a nice walk and people watching along the plaza. It is a good distraction from my fatigue. Ines shares her experience with her father during the days prior to his passing from lung cancer. It makes me sad as I wonder what my fate will be.

....

Friday, July 26

Scott and I leave for Zug, Switzerland, today to see my friend and coworker Dean, his wife Cherie, and their children, Nathan, Jacob and Eryn. We're scheduled to leave at 11 AM. Scott and I love traveling by train versus driving. It's stressful driving in a foreign country. We've driven a few times on previous European trips.

Having done so, we prefer traveling by train. It's fun and more adventurous. Unfortunately, our three-and-a-half-hour train ride turns into six hours due to excessive heat that causes trains to be delayed. The Swiss are very punctual. If a train is late, they won't think twice about re-routing your train. This is exactly what they do. Our stop in Zug is eliminated; we have no choice but to get off as close as possible to Zug, which ends up being about twenty miles west of the town. We are prepared to take a taxi back to Zug, but Cherie and Dean won't have it. They come to pick us up. It is wonderful seeing them. We look forward to our time together. Scott and I have no expectations. We're perfectly content to make our stay simple. We rarely stay with friends so as to be less of a burden.

Saturday, July 27

Scott and I enjoy some much-needed down time with Cherie and Dean. We plan a trip to Weggis, Switzerland, a charming town nearby on Lake Lucerne, to have lunch, our treat. We end up at Oliv, a very nice restaurant with table seating on a terrace overlooking the picturesque lake. The sun is glistening on the water. It's a magnificent day. What a great way to start our visit with our dear friends. Their son, Nathan, joins us. We enjoy our lunch as we continue to bask in the sunlight. It rains later in the afternoon, so we get cozy on the sofa and settle in to binge-watch a Netflix sci-fi series.

Sunday, July 28

The rain continues today. Scott and I slept in Jacob's room. Jacob generously gave up his room and slept in the second single bed in Nathan's room. We barely see Jacob during our stay. He's spending time with his friends, enjoying his last summer before starting his senior year in high school. Scott and I totally understand,

and we smile at each other as we each think of our last summer before starting our senior year in high school. Nathan is fourteen years old. He's smart and always very respectful to his parents. He's the best kid ever!

Tired of being indoors, Cherie and Dean find a castle for us to visit. We spend the afternoon at Wildegg Castle, about an hour away. The castle was built around 1242 by the royal Habsburgs, though upon completion they never lived there. The castle is totally cool. There are digital interactive historic overviews for each room. Afterward, there is a falconer who conducts a wonderful demonstration with owls and falcons!

Monday, July 29

Cherie and Nathan drop us off at the Zug train station. Scott and I travel to nearby Lucerne to spend the day sightseeing. We enjoy a leisurely lunch at an outside café located along the water, next to the Chapel Bridge. It's a cloudy, breezy day with temperatures around 72°F. We walk over five miles around the city and visit the beautiful granite sculpture Lion Monument. We stop at Heini Conditorei in downtown Lucerne. They are widely known for their delicious cherry liqueur–filled chocolates. The chocolates are made right there in the store. We have fun choosing a large gift box of these chocolates as our gift to Cherie and Dean, our wonderful friends and gracious hosts.

We meet Dean after work. He works nearby at the MSD (Merck) office in Lucerne. Together we take the train back to Zug. Dean and Cherie have arranged a special dinner on our last night. We will be eating at Fischmärt, a nearby local Italian restaurant. Eryn is back from a trip to Prague with some college friends who were visiting from the U.S. over their summer college break. We're happy to see Eryn here in Zug with her family before she heads back to school.

Dean and Cherie open our gifts. The Heini Conditorei chocolates along with a bottle of Veuve Clicquot champagne are well received. We enjoy a toast, and a piece of delicious chocolate, before leaving for dinner. Scott and I enjoy a lovely dinner with our dear friends at a large rectangular table just outside the restaurant in the cobblestone courtyard. Cherie and Dean have been wonderful hosts, very kind, very thoughtful and very generous. Scott and I will cherish the memory of this trip always.

Tuesday, July 30

It's difficult saying goodbye to Cherie before leaving for the airport. She's so loving. Dean graciously drives us to the Zurich airport. We're happy that Eryn comes along. They both walk us right up to the International Security checkpoint. As with Cherie, it's hard to say goodbye to Dean and Eryn. Scott and I are grateful to have such wonderful friends. I have tears in my eyes as I hug them both, already wondering when or if I will see them again.

Our flight back to the States is uneventful. We arrive at Newark Airport late in the afternoon and spend at least an hour in line at U.S. Customs. At this point, I am in pain. My back hurts from standing so long. This is most likely due to the five miles we walked yesterday in Lucerne coupled with sitting seven hours on our long flight home. It is a bit unbearable. Scott and I decide that next time we travel internationally we will arrange for me to have a wheelchair.

Wednesday, July 31

Scott and I are jet-lagged today. We expected this based on our previous trips. I wake up with some pain on the left side of my pelvis but decline to take any pain meds. The pain dissipates by bedtime.

August

....

Thursday, August 1

Today I have my second appointment with Dr. Langer. This is the first time we have seen each other since my MRI and CT scans at the beginning of July. Dr. Langer is very pleased with the results of my scans. He is happy that my brain tumors are gone and that my lymph nodes and primary tumor have shrunk. He confirms that I am in remission with a partial response of 50 percent or greater tumor burden reduction.

As with my first appointment, Dr. Langer and I review the various clinical studies: Pointbreak and Empower 150. Both studies use Avastin. Additionally, he shares an ongoing investigator-driven extension of Keynote-189. It's a small phase 2 study. The investigator is using Pemetrexed, carboplatin and Avastin, plus or minus Keytruda, from a sampling of patients with high PD-L1 who are EGFR positive. Dr. Langer also reviews Keynote-001, which had a five-year update presented at this year's ASCO conference. Although this is a single-agent study, Dr. Langer associates my progress with those patients at the top of the Kaplan-Meier curve.[28] These are the patients with the highest survival benefit.

Dr. Langer is happy to hear that Scott and I had a good time on our trip. He reinforces how important it is to continue to "live" regardless of having lung cancer. Every time I see Dr. Langer, I feel energized with confidence that I just might beat this. After today's visit, I know I will.

[28.] The Kaplan-Meier curve is used to estimate the survival function. The visual representation of this function is usually called the Kaplan-Meier curve, and it shows what the probability of an event (for example, survival) is at a certain time interval. *Source: https://www.ncbi.nlm.nih.gov/pmc/articles/PMC3059453/*

Friday, August 2

Today I receive my fourth cycle of Keytruda Combo. All goes well. This is the last planned treatment cycle dose that includes carboplatin.

My pre-treatment blood work shows that my liver enzymes are good. My July 12 results show my AST at 19, down from 28; and my ALT at 18, down from 41. My alkaline phosphatase clocks in at 390, down from 461.

My red blood cell (RBC) count is 3.57 (range: 4.60-6.20); hemoglobin is 9.8 (range: 10.0-14.0); and hematocrit is 31.6 (range: 42-52) These low red blood cell counts are typical with chemotherapy.

My next CT scan is confirmed. It is scheduled at the Blue Bell, Pennsylvania, Abington-Jefferson Radiology Center on Monday, August 19.

Saturday, August 3

I feel good today relative to how I typically feel one day after my cycle. My overall fatigue isn't as bad. My discomfort and pain are minimal. I take a mid-afternoon nap. This helps. Today is my last day of dexamethasone day-after, post-cycle treatment dose. I'm back to practicing my horn daily. It's good to be back after a much-needed vacation.

Sunday, August 4

At noon, I begin to come down from my nadir. Fatigue sets in as expected, though my overall fatigue isn't as bad as it was post first, second and third cycles.

Monday, August 5

I get through the night without any night sweats. I've been having night sweats over the past month. There's no fever. I just sweat a lot. I believe this is my body shedding the cancer.

My fatigue, however, sets in and I end up having to take two nap breaks this afternoon. I've been working from home on Mondays, Tuesdays and Fridays; going into the office on Wednesdays and Thursdays. This schedule has been working well since early July, though I am nauseous today. The nausea sets in around 7 PM. I take half a Compazine dose, 5 mg, at 7 PM and the other half at bedtime. This helps, and I have a good night's sleep.

Tuesday, August 6

I have less fatigue today. My overall strength is returning as per usual during this same time period subsequent to cycle treatments. My nausea is mild. Scott has developed flu-like symptoms.

Wednesday, August 7

It's official, Scott has a cold and so do I. Damn! Fatigue is back and I am congested. On top of fighting the cancer, I feel my immune system pulling double-duty to fight off the cold. I hang in there and go into the office due to some meetings I want to attend in-person. I develop chills in the afternoon, and my energy level decreases even more. It's raining, which doesn't help. Luckily, I have an umbrella, though this doesn't help with my chills as I walk to my car in the parking garage. I make it home and immediately take a two-hour nap. This is my second-worst fatigue day since the last week of June. It's similar to how I felt after my bronchoscopy in May. I am hit hard.

I wake up from my nap with a fever and feel nauseous. I'm drinking lots of water. The nausea subsides a bit so that by 7 PM I have a sandwich and begin to feel better. I wear long underwear to bed to help manage and avoid more chills.

Thursday, August 8

I sleep well, though my cold and congestion continue. My fatigue is greater than it was during the same time period after my third cycle. I believe this is due to my cold. I still go into the office for several in-person meetings. I know, I'm crazy. Somehow working serves as a good distraction from my cancer. It also helps me feel like I still have a "normal" life. Unfortunately, I develop chills again in the afternoon. The air-conditioning doesn't help. They keep it cool in the office during the summertime, which makes sense. Thank goodness that Scott is with me. I asked him to come to work with me today to provide support. This helps a lot! It's comforting having him with me. Work colleagues who recognize Scott are very kind and supportive. He fits in well with the Merck culture. I couldn't have gotten through my workday without him. My chills subside later in the afternoon. We return home and I take a nap. This time it's only an hour. I feel much better when I wake up, though nausea has haunted me again today. As I've done before, I take half of a Compazine, 5 mg, at 4 PM and the other half at bedtime.

Friday, August 9

My cold and congestion continue today, though it seems to be clearing. Like clockwork, my chills return in the afternoon followed by nausea. Fortunately, I'm working from home today. I take a mid-afternoon nap and feel better. I love naps! I always feel better after a nap. Once again, I take split doses of Compazine, and I drink lots of water. This seems to be helping. Fortunately, I'm not experiencing any discomfort or pain this week. My body is able to focus on recovering from my cold.

I can tell Keytruda Combo is working by the sensation (feeling) of heat radiating from my skin in the areas where there are lymph nodes. I usually notice this in the early evening. On this day, there are more than a few areas radiating heat versus one or two.

I go to bed and wake up at 2:30 AM sopping wet. I am literally sleeping in a puddle of water. What is this all about? The sheets around me, my pillows and my PJs are all soaking wet. Despite being wet, I feel good. I immediately change into dry clothes and replace my pillow. Fortunately, I don't wake up Scott. However strange this experience is, I truly believe there was a lot of cancer killed tonight. I've experienced night sweats before, but they were nothing compared to this. If my prior sweat experiences could be characterized as a chamber string quartet, this time it was a full-blown symphony orchestra!

Saturday, August 10

I wake up feeling good and try to understand what I went through last night. I would have called my doctor had I not awoken feeling well. Last night's experience amazes me. Scott and I head to our clubhouse for a swim. We like to go early in the morning before anyone gets there. We do this weekly. We enjoy our time together at the pool. I don't swim much. I usually do my laps by walking briskly back and forth through the water from end to end. I really like the jacuzzi. It's very refreshing early in the morning with the sun shining.

Scott and I spend the afternoon out and about. We enjoy our day together. His birthday is tomorrow. We have dinner reservations tonight at the Blue Bell Inn. It's been awhile since we were last there. We arrive and enjoy a Venetian Spritz before appetizers. Our dinner is good. I'm really not feeling well today, but my desire to be with Scott to celebrate his birthday overrides everything.

Sunday, August 11

Today is Scott's birthday—yeah! I get up early and head out to Starbucks. Scott started doing this for my birthday years ago. It took me a few years to catch on. It's a bright, sunny day as I drive to get coffee. For the first day since earlier in the week, I don't have chills during the afternoon. I'm not sure if Scott's birthday has anything to do with this, but I'll take it! We enjoy a wonderful day together. Scott has had a great year. He works very hard and is always there for me. I am very proud of him. Together, we can do anything!

Monday, August 12

Today is a good day. My congestion seems to be breaking up. My breathing is easier. I continue my schedule of working at home part of the week. This is my first, good quality day in over a week. I have more strength with no fatigue. My nausea is gone. I have a good horn rehearsal. I can feel that my lungs are clearer.

Tuesday, August 13

It's raining today. We needed the rain. I continue to feel good with some lingering congestion. My chills and nausea are gone. Scott and I continue to walk at least 1.5 miles per day.

Wednesday-Friday, August 14-16

Each day I wake up feeling stronger. I have some night sweats but wake up with more energy each day. I go into the office and stay until the end of the day. My day is very productive. My energy doesn't dip in the afternoon as it has before. My appetite is good with no chills and no nausea. Horn practice goes well. It's been a good week.

Saturday, August 17

I'm glad it's the weekend. Scott and I run some errands. My energy level continues to improve. We have lunch in downtown

Skippack. I am able to sit in a chair that is somewhat uncomfortable. No problem though; there's no back pain. This would not have happened back in early May. The back pain would have been unbearable. Today I didn't even need a cushion for back support!

Scott and I set the date for our Celebration of Life, Love and Friendship party. It will be Saturday afternoon, November 16. We want to thank our friends for all of their support. It is very important to take the opportunity to acknowledge all of their love and support. These are our friends and family of choice. Their unconditional love and support mean the world to Scott and me.

My horn rehearsal goes well. My ability to move between registers has improved. I can't remember playing like this before. My lungs feel good. I have no pain or discomfort. I'm relaxed and can feel my endurance building.

§

I was in seventh grade when I first started playing the French horn. I wanted to play the trumpet like my dad did when he was in junior high. Unfortunately, there were too many other kids also interested and there were only six trumpets. To be fair, our band teacher wrote "trumpet," along with "euphonium," "trombone" and "French horn" on pieces of paper. Everyone had to pick one. You got it, I picked the French horn, or maybe the French horn picked me! I practiced all the time. At first, it sounded like a dying moose! Year by year, I got better. One of my fondest memories is when I was home from college one weekend preparing for my junior recital. I was practicing the Mozart Concerto no. 3 in E-flat Major, K. 447. My mom, who was always very quiet and never commented on my playing—yes, even when it sounded like a moose in distress—started humming the horn melody from the concerto. She shared with me how much she liked my playing. We laughed together as we reminisced about those early days when I was learning to play. It's a memory I cherish. If I had to give a single reason for why I returned to playing the horn after so many years, that special moment with my mom would be the one.

....

Sunday, August 18

I had a good night, though the night sweats have returned. Nothing too bad though. My energy is good, with no nausea. Scott and I go to the clubhouse to swim and use the jacuzzi. It's so early, we have the pool and jacuzzi to ourselves. Afterward, we run some errands.

I've been thinking about my CT scan appointment tomorrow. Scott and I wonder how much progress I may have made since my last CT scan at the beginning of July. We continue to be positive with our thoughts and hold onto the belief that the finish line is in sight. We're hoping to have 80 percent of the cancer gone. We base this on how I've been feeling, especially over the past few weeks. The only daily medication I'm taking other than my cancer treatment is folic acid, Xarelto and an Ambien PRN (as needed) at night. My cancer treatments are every three weeks. We are very happy that I'm pain-free and feeling better every day.

....

Monday, August 19

Today is another good day! I'm ready for my next CT scan at the Abington-Jefferson Blue Bell radiation building. This scan is eighty days post–initial treatment. (My July scan was thirty-five days post-treatment, and 50 percent of my cancer was gone based on the results then.) This time Scott and I believe that my primary tumor and lymph nodes have shrunk dramatically. We also believe the lesions on my spine are gone or near gone. My appetite is very good. It's so good that Scott and I stop and get an Italian hoagie on our way home. We haven't done this in a while. We enjoy lunch and a long afternoon nap afterward.

Tuesday, August 20

I'm feeling so much better now that I decide to go into the office for several face-to-face meetings. I am able to sit at my desk with no cushion behind my back. I'm not experiencing any discomfort. I am anxious to hear about the results from my third CT scan, but there's no word today. Hopefully, I'll hear something tomorrow. I wonder if the results will be from baseline when I had my very first CT scan in May or from where I was at on July 5.

Wednesday, August 21

Dr. CO calls in the afternoon to share the results of my CT scan. She starts our conversation by asking me how I feel. "Great!" I say, and share that I feel the most "normal" I've felt since I was diagnosed with cancer. I have no pain, no fatigue and no nausea.

Dr. CO tells me that my cancer has either shrunk or is gone. No cancer was detected in my pelvis and supraclavicular areas. My primary lower lung tumor has been reduced in size from a grape to a raisin—it's now 2.5×2.0 cm—and all previously detected lymph nodes with cancer have been reduced to around 9 mm. There are no lesions on my spine, either. This accounts for the reduction of back pain. This is the best day ever since my cancer diagnosis!

Thursday, August 22

This is the day before my first maintenance dose of Keytruda/Alimta begins. No more carboplatin per the treatment protocol defined and used in Keynote-189. This will be my fifth cycle of treatment. I feel great! No fatigue, no nausea and absolutely no pain.

Friday, August 23

Scott and I arrive at the Asplundh Cancer Center early. We meet with Dr. CO, who reviews the CT scan images, comparing them to my May 15 baseline images. It is stunning to see how much cancer is gone! I'm excited to be starting the maintenance dosing of Keytruda/Alimta.

Saturday, August 24

I'm feeling good today, the day after receiving my Keytruda/Alimta maintenance dose. There's no fatigue or nausea.

Sunday, August 25

I'm still not feeling any fatigue or nausea today. This is contrary to how I felt after my previous four Keytruda Combo cycles, each containing Keytruda, Alimta and carboplatin. I feel good.

Monday, August 26

Today, I wake up feeling fatigued. I end up having to take a two-hour nap from noon until 2 PM and another from 4 to 5 PM. I feel much better after my second nap.

Tuesday, August 27

My fatigue continues, but is better than it was on Monday. I continue to rest appropriately. I experience no nausea or sensitivity to cold. Scott and I keep up our daily walks.

Wednesday, August 28

I'm feeling less fatigued today. I'm able to go into the office, as planned. I develop a muscle spasm in my upper left rib area. There is some pain. I was coughing when this occurred. I have been coughing up clear fluid Dr. Langer likes to call "schmutz." This is a Yiddish word that describes an unpleasant substance—in other words, a fancy word for "dirt." I'm still only taking Xarelto and folic acid in the morning and Ambien at night. I haven't taken any pain meds for about two months now. My appetite continues to be good. I've had very little change in my weight, maintaining 170 pounds since my diagnosis.

Thursday, August 29

My left rib spasm is beginning to feel better. I decide to use a Diclofenac Epolamine pain patch on the area, which provides the relief I was looking for. I only feel discomfort when I cough, otherwise I feel good.

Friday, August 30

My left rib spasm is better, and I no longer need to use the topical patch. Despite this, I go to work. I was asked by senior leadership to share my lung cancer journey with a good-sized group of new hires at a local conference center in Blue Bell. Our Merck physician patient advocate, my friend Dr. Linda, is there to ask questions and guide me through my story. I'm glad that she's on stage with me. All goes well, the group is very supportive, though I must admit that it is tough reliving my journey. Especially since this is the first time I've shared my journey, out loud, in front of a lot of people, most of whom I haven't met before.

My schmutz has decreased. I'm able to continue practicing my horn playing. I took a few days off so as not to overdo the use of my lungs given the spasm on my left side. I immediately notice improvement in my playing. I'm able to control my breathing better than I have in a long time. This makes me happy.

Saturday, August 31

Despite tightness in my left rib area, I'm feeling better with little or no fatigue. Scott and I are invited to a friend's home to celebrate Labor Day weekend. We have a wonderful time during our visit.

SEPTEMBER

....

Sunday–Monday, September 1–2

We continue to enjoy our Labor Day weekend. My rib spasm continues to subside. It's a beautiful day! Scott and I enjoy a two-mile walk on the nearby Perkiomen Trail and spend the rest of the holiday weekend resting and watching movies. It is very relaxing.

....

Tuesday, September 3

I have an appointment with Dr. Langer at Penn Medicine today. This is my third appointment with Dr. Langer. My last appointment was at the beginning of August. Dr. Langer has my previous CT scans on disc from Abington-Jefferson and compares my August results with my baseline scan from May. He points out areas where the cancer has shrunk dramatically or is gone. He confirms that I have had a "strong" response. It's official: I am in partial response. Dr. Langer says 75 to 80 percent of my cancer is gone. The finish line is near!

Scott and I do the Scooby dance afterward. I think about the day I was diagnosed, three and one-half months ago. I hear the fourth movement from Beethoven's Symphony no. 5 in my head.[29] After introducing a gloom-and-doom

29. *Music*: Beethoven Symphony no. 5 in C Minor, op. 67 and Beethoven Symphony no. 6 in F Major, op. 68. Yannick Nézet-Séguin and the Philadelphia Orchestra BeethovenNow Concert Series, March 2020 performance (YouTube video, 1:26:35). Minute 31:27 marks the beginning of the fourth movement of Beethoven Symphony no. 5 in C Minor, op. 67. Posted by the Philadelphia Orchestra, March 14, 2020; accessed September 2020. *https://www.youtube.com/watch?v=zKWYX5ohadQ*

opening in his famous first movement of the 5th Symphony, here in the last movement Beethoven introduces a melody that seems to sing a message of rejoicing. It reinforces my belief that behind every tragic or challenging event there is an opposite feeling of magnificence waiting for us. The soft murmur in the beginning of the last movement seems to go on forever before exploding into a big beautiful sound; it perfectly depicts how I'm feeling today and my thoughts of being cancer free.

Wednesday, September 4

I'm feeling the best ever since I started my journey! This is what Scott and I envisioned. As I've said, when I was first diagnosed, I had severe back pain. Since my initial histology provided the information we needed to start my first treatment, I decided, based on my pain, to begin with Keytruda Combo. We went with what we knew at that time. Considering how I feel today, I stand by this decision. Here I am with 80 percent of my cancer gone. This is absolutely incredible! There is so much we still don't know about the potential of Keytruda. I am a living testimony. Tagrisso will continue to be my Plan B if and when the cancer begins to grow again.

Playing my French horn continues to be a great indicator for me as to how I am doing. This evening I can feel a noticeable improvement in my horn playing. I am able to breath deeper, with more control. My breathing is sustained, and my endurance is getting better each day. This is evident as I play the horn solo excerpts from Beethoven's 6th Symphony. My sound is free and flowing. The high notes are relaxed and very melodic, as though they were plucked out of thin air.

Friday, September 6

I suddenly wake up around 4 AM with severe pain on the left side of my lower back. Not sure why. I haven't felt this type of pain since mid-July. I take an Advil and am able to go back to sleep. I let Scott know as soon as we wake up together at 7 AM. We are worried. I apply a Diclofenac Epolamine pain patch, but it doesn't seem to work. The pain is so severe I need to take an Aleve and 800 mg of Metaxalone; that combination works a little. I have a hard time typing on the computer. Any slight movement forward in my chair causes severe pain and nausea. I consider going to the hospital, but the very thought of going on a stronger pain med like morphine or oxycodone rules that out. It's so bad that I am panting. I even apply an ice pack directly to the pain area. Fortunately, over the next hour, the pain subsides. By 3 PM, the pain is more manageable, and I am able to feel some comfort. My nausea was really bad in the morning and that also subsides in the afternoon.

Scott is very concerned at the sudden reoccurrence of severe pain. Both of us are frustrated. He goes to get lunch for us when I start feeling better. It is a very large sandwich, which sounds good, but I am so hungry that I eat too much, and this then causes me to be sick to my stomach with indigestion. I am so upset.

Scott has been so wonderful throughout my journey, even more so today. I can't imagine what it must be like, from his point of view, to see me in so much pain and discomfort. I can see the worry on his face. Scott isn't as expressive as I am. Seeing him this way is upsetting. He offers multiple ideas to help me feel better. He's always so good at asking me what he can do and never complains. It makes me sad to see him worry. Scott is wonderful! I want to get better so we can continue our life together.

This is a tough, emotional day for us. For all that we've been through, up until this point, having achieved 80 percent of the cancer being gone or shrunk, how can I be experiencing this level of pain out of the blue? What has changed? What is going on? We want this cancer gone so badly. I want my life back. I am not dying of lung cancer. I want to live. This is not acceptable. It needs to stop now! Echoes of the foreboding first movement of Beethoven's 5th Symphony return and play continuously in my head.[30]

The bizarre day brings one piece of good news though; the coughing and schmutz have stopped. It seems as though a trade-off has occurred. I wish I could feel better about that, but all I can think is: *Please. No. More. Pain.*

Saturday, September 7

I wake up feeling better than I did yesterday. Thank goodness! My pain has subsided. Because of the pain medication I took, I am now constipated. This makes me uncomfortable. I have mild nausea. Despite this, Scott and I walk 3.1 miles on the Perkiomen Trail. It is a beautiful day. Cancer can kiss my ass!

Sunday, September 8

I feel about the same today as I did yesterday. I still have some pain and discomfort. I'm still constipated and continue to have moderate nausea. I take a laxative and hope it works soon. Bloating, as you may know, is a very uncomfortable feeling to have. I take it easy today and only walk 1.2 miles.

I play my French horn and manage to have a good practice. I play the Beethoven Trio, op. 81b, first movement, along with the

---

[30.] *Music:* Beethoven Symphony no. 5 in C Minor, op. 67 and Beethoven Symphony no. 6 in F Major, op. 68. Yannick Nézet-Séguin and the Philadelphia Orchestra BeethovenNow Concert Series, March 2020 performance (YouTube video, 1:26:35). Symphony no. 5 begins at minute 10:37. It is proceeded by the opening performance of Habibi's "Jeder Baum spricht." Posted by the Philadelphia Orchestra, March 14, 2020; accessed September 2020. *https://www.youtube.com/watch?v=zKWYX5ohadQ*

Beethoven Horn Sonata, op. 17. I don't have cancer when I play my horn.

....

Monday, September 9

I'm hanging in there, feeling about the same as I did over the weekend. I finally have a bowel movement and feel better right away. My pain and discomfort are holding at a six on a scale of ten. Despite this, I work all day from home and feel good enough to go on a long walk at the end of the day, 2.4 miles on the Perkiomen Trail. The weather is cooler now, approaching a new sunset as autumn draws near. The air quality feels noticeably better.

During our walk, as we are crossing the footbridge, my husband looks down and sees a large turtle underwater. Since the sex is unknown, we'll refer to this turtle as "they." We watch in amazement as they move under the bridge. Once under, the turtle makes their way toward the shore, where they come up for air. This turtle is an awesome sight to watch. It is large; it appears to be at least four feet in length with a thick neck. Its head and tail, extending in either direction out of the shell, make it seem even longer. The shell has markings and arches high from its base. It's magnificent to watch while we debate how old this turtle must be. We think that they're at least 80 years old based on its size. What a beautiful turtle!

....

Tuesday, September 10

I'm beginning to feel better. I'm becoming more regular as my bowel movements are improving. My pain and discomfort are okay. Pain comes and goes. When it comes, it's sharp and then after about an hour it suddenly goes away. An hour later, it's back. What is up with this? Scott and I aren't sure if this is cancer related or a side effect.

Wednesday, September 11

I continue to feel better. My pain and discomfort continue to decrease. Scott and I hope these days of returning pain go away completely soon. We diligently continue with our walks. I think about what happened eighteen years ago today. I am sad as I reflect on all those who lost their lives on 9/11 in 2001. I am reminded how precious life is. I am grateful to still be here. I mourn for our fallen citizens and wonder what lies ahead for me.

Thursday, September 12

We're not sure what this last pain episode was, but Scott and I remain optimistic that it was nothing more than a speed bump. I'm regular now and have little or no nausea and fatigue. I continue to feel better and believe this cancer is going away and the finish line is within sight. Giddy-up!

Friday, September 13

Today I have my second Keytruda/Alimta maintenance cycle dose scheduled. This is my sixth cycle overall. My bowel movements are normal, and my pain and discomfort are minimal. Overall, my energy level has improved coming into this next treatment cycle.

Scott and I meet with Dr. CO prior to treatment. Our meeting goes well. We discuss my current trajectory of improvement given the relatively short amount of time since starting treatment, including when a complete response might occur. Dr. CO believes a complete response may occur and, based on my current trajectory, agrees that it could occur prior to the next scan. The next scan is scheduled to be completed the week of November 11. We put all our positive energy toward this thought. It's not a matter of *if*, it's *when!*

Saturday, September 14

We are happy that it's the weekend! The weather is perfect! Scott and I take advantage of the nice weather and walk 2.7 miles. We reminisce about our college days and the years before we met. We begin planning for my birthday: April 22, 2020. The decision is made to spend my sixtieth birthday in Venice. Scott and I have spent several birthdays there—all of them memorable—with our "Venetian family." We are excited to return to Venice, especially since we couldn't make it there this past summer due to my cancer.

We first met our Venetian friend Alessandro in 1997. He was our gondolier for our first Venetian gondola ride. Since then, we've gone back to Venice almost every year. Each visit, we get to know Alessandro, his wife Alessandra and their families, better. Together, we explore the beautiful, timeless city of Venice. During our trip, we plan to spend ten days in Venice, leaving on April 29 for Paris. We make a very big decision: to take the Belmond Orient Express train from Venice to Paris. We decide to splurge and book a Grand Parlor Suite, especially since it is the only compartment that has its own bath and shower. Aside from the three Grand Parlor Suites on each Orient Express train, all other compartments are much smaller and only have a sink. They share a common toilet in each car, none of which have a shower. It's a lot of money for the suite, but it will be worth it. You only live once.

Sunday, September 15

I'm feeling better. Scott and I enjoy a long walk today. The weather is beautiful, cool with a light breeze, low humidity and good air quality. After our walk, we continue our plans for my sixtieth birthday trip. It's nice to plan something. Over these last months, I've seen my future through a short-term lens: day by day and week by week. I haven't wanted to overwhelm or pressure myself to be at a certain point by a certain date or time. The future has been uncertain. I remember when only about half of lung cancer patients made it through their first year.

Now I begin to realize what I've known all along: I am beating this. I am winning my battle with lung cancer. I remember my first words to Dr. Steve the day he told me I had cancer: "This is not how I'm going to die."

Monday, September 16

I'm working from home today, as I continue to do every Monday. I feel my nadir hit around 2 PM as fatigue sets in. It is mild compared to how I felt after my Keytruda Combo treatment cycles when carboplatin was included. Without carboplatin my side effects are mild. I take my afternoon nap and feel good when I wake up. I decide to take a break from horn rehearsal today and choose to take a walk with Scott instead. I grow tired around 9 PM, which typically does not happen. It's okay though since it's close to bedtime. Overall, my nadir is manageable.

Tuesday, September 17

My day-after treatment symptoms are good overall as compared to other Tuesdays after previous treatments. My fatigue is mild with very little nausea. Scott can tell I am feeling better when I playfully stick my tongue out at him as I walk by him in the morning. I used to do this every now and then just for fun. Scott roars with laughter as he realizes that it's been a while since I last did this. He knows I'm getting better. I actually told Scott that I was going to include this in my book. So, here it is! 😛

Wednesday, September 18

I go to work today. I always look forward to my days in the office. With all that I'm going through, I continue to enjoy working and seeing my coworkers. My overall energy level continues to improve. The feeling of disconnect or fogginess has diminished. I continue to be hopeful that I'll achieve a complete response soon.

....

Thursday, September 19

I continue to sleep well. The occasional nighttime restlessness I experienced when carboplatin was part of my regimen is gone. I do not feel as tired in the afternoon as I did yesterday. My overall energy level has improved. I realize that I haven't received an automated email from Abington-Jefferson indicating my lab results have been uploaded, so I log in to my patient portal to check. Blood continues to be drawn before each treatment cycle. I completed my sixth treatment cycle last Friday, September 13. Luckily, several lab results from that date have been uploaded. My alkaline phosphatase is now 242, down from 380 on August 23.[31] As a point of reference, I look up my alkaline phosphatase before I was diagnosed. On March 16 of this year, it was 67, and on April 9 it was 65. On May 14, it rose to 186. On June 23 it was 403. On July 12, it hit 461. Then in August, it began declining: 390 on August 2, and 380 on August 23. I remember that alkaline phosphatase is said to be a positive prognostic indicator of cancer remission. When it was in the 400s in July and August, I asked Dr. CO if we should be concerned about this and was told "No, it is part of the cancer." So now that my alkaline phosphatase is dropping, along with my overall quality of life improving, Scott and I are looking at this as a very positive sign that the cancer is going away.

....

Friday, September 20

I wake up feeling good this morning. I have a very productive day working from home. One of the measurements I use to gauge how

---

[31.] As a reminder, ALK phosphatase normal range is 40-150.

I feel is making the bed. I look at this as exercise. In the past, when I was first diagnosed with metastatic non–small cell lung cancer, it would take at least forty-five minutes to make the bed. Today, it takes less than fifteen minutes! And I no longer need any breaks!

Because I'm feeling better, I've been able to increase my daily walking to over two miles. My legs feel stronger. I follow Dr. Langer's advice not to do weight training so that I don't over-exert myself while my lymph nodes and cancer continue to shrink. Scott and I continue to swim most weekends at the club-house. We enjoy our time together there in the water along with the nice weather. The jacuzzi usually takes thirty minutes to heat up, which is inconvenient, but once it's hot enough it feels great!

Saturday, September 21

Scott and I are going to my hometown of Scranton, Pennsylvania, this afternoon to see my Uncle Jimmy. I am able to fit in a horn practice before we leave, in preparation for my horn lesson with Jack tomorrow at Curtis Institute. Uncle Jimmy is my mom's only living sibling. He is age seventy-seven with a birthday coming up in October. He has a son, Jimmy Jr., along with three grandchil-dren: Dominique, Jaimi and Jordan, and five great-grandchildren: Valland, Azlyn, Lael, Julia and River. During our visit, we are delighted to meet them at Jimmy Jr. and his wife Michelle's home. They have a lovely home and made a beautiful life for themselves. I'm happy to see my cousin Jimmy Jr. again. It's been at least thirty-five years since we last saw each other. Uncle Jimmy is a good guy. You can tell that he is my mom's brother. He is very pos-itive and genuinely supports Scott and me.

Although we are enjoying our visit, it's always difficult for me to go back home to Scranton. My childhood memories are happy ones, but as a teenager, most of them are not very good. Going back home is like going back in time for me. I prefer to live my life in the present, always moving forward. Before we leave town, we stop at

Cathedral Cemetery to visit Jimmy's late wife, my Aunt Micky. "Micky" is short for Michelina. A beautiful name for a beautiful person. Uncle Jimmy and Aunt Micky were married over fifty-five years. She was a great lady who had a beautiful smile every time I saw her. Aunt Micky rests in front of my grandparents, Rachel and Dominic. Sadly, after years of fighting metastatic melanoma, Aunt Micky passed away in November 2018. This is the main reason I decide not to tell my Uncle Jimmy about my lung cancer. We also visit my mom, who is buried alongside her mom and dad. It's been a while since my last visit. I take a moment by myself at her gravesite to tell her that I know she's with me and thank her for being there.

Scott and I then head to the Bellevue Hotel in downtown Philadelphia. We enjoy our stays there. Aside from my horn lesson tomorrow afternoon, we will be attending an evening Philadelphia Orchestra performance of Dvořák's 9th Symphony, "From the New World." We always enjoy going to Philadelphia Orchestra concerts. We're looking forward to tonight's performance. Scott and I are very excited as this is the first time we will hear this symphony performed live. The performance is awesome! Jack walks up the aisle at intermission, right to where Scott and I are sitting. I didn't realize he would be here. We meet afterward for drinks at the Ritz Carlton. We recap the performance and I share with Jack that I'm able to play the fourth movement horn solo from Beethoven's Symphony no. 6 better now and how happy I am, given my journey. I don't remember my playing being so free and easy compared to how it was in college.

Sunday, September 22

Today, I resume my horn lessons with Jack. This will be the first lesson as Louis 2.0 since our Curtis Summerfest performance. My horn lesson goes well—the best ever! I play all of Kopprasch Study no. 13 for Jack. After I finish, Jack sits back in his chair and expresses amazement at how well I sound. He says it is the best he's heard me play, a full sound that is strong. I smile as I think to myself: *That's Louis 2.0 playing.* I let Jack know that my lungs are functioning better and my physical therapy of playing the French horn is working. It's my best barometer for how I am feeling.

I truly believe that playing my French horn is saving my life.

Monday, September 23

I haven't felt any nausea or pain discomfort for just over a week now. I do grow tired in the afternoon and take a nap. Scott and I take our daily walk. I have a good horn practice session. I apply the breathing tips Jack gave me during my lesson, and they work! I am on a good path now with my horn playing. The quality and accuracy of my sound mirrors how I feel. What better way of knowing my metastatic non-small cell lung cancer is going away than having the ability to play the French horn better and more beautifully! 😄

Tuesday, September 24

I think I may have spoken too soon. This morning I wake up with discomfort similar to the pain I felt a couple weeks ago. This time the pain is centered on my lower left side. Despite how I'm feeling, I go into the office. I have a thirty-minute meeting at 2:30 PM that I want to be in-person for. I feel bloated. I'm not sure if this pain is related to the cancer or constipation. After my meeting, I leave to work from home. The pain increases as I walk to my car. I'm panting from the pain as I sit in my car. The pain continues to increase after dinner. I believe that my daily dose of two Senokot-S in the morning is not working. I take two Dulcolax tablets at bedtime along with one Advil. This is the first time I can remember taking anything for pain in a while, due to the potential damage to my liver. I feel relief right away so that I'm able to relax and fall asleep. I awake at 2 AM feeling better.

I don't recall feeling any pain, discomfort or diarrhea during the second week of my cycle. Perhaps something has changed? Is there something like stomach bacteria causing my constipation? Is my pain related to constipation or cancer? These are questions I will be asking Dr. CO when I go in for my seventh Keytruda/Alimta maintenance cycle next Friday.

Wednesday, September 25

I have a bowel movement this morning and instantly feel better. My energy level is good, and I'm able to go into the office. The day goes well, though toward mid-afternoon I begin to feel some back pain. After dinner the bloating returns, along with some nausea. My pain increases as it did yesterday and continues into the evening. I take two Dulcolax and one Advil, same as yesterday, and have a good night's sleep. Scott and I continue to walk two miles a day. We believe that my discomfort may be related to the increased physical activity. Maybe the cancer does not like that. Perhaps my physical activity is causing the cancer to come out from hiding. It feels like Keytruda has jump-started my immune system so that my body can go after the cancer and kill it. In the past, whenever I experienced this kind of pain and discomfort, it has always led to shrinking of the cancer or having the cancer be gone in areas such as my lymph nodes.

Thursday, September 26

I wake up feeling better. I am regular and my back pain has decreased. I've noticed over the past three days that I've been experiencing a pinched nerve-type sensation down my left side into my calf. This is the leg where DVT was discovered. I wonder if the pain on my left side where the primary tumor is located has anything to do with this. It's more annoying than anything. Despite this, Scott and I walk tonight believing that physical activity can only help.

Friday, September 27

I continue to feel better. Thank goodness! My back pain is minimal now. I go into the office again today. This is the first Friday I've gone into the office since before my cancer was discovered. I have a good day but again, my back pain increases as the day goes on. Perhaps I'm overexerting myself? This is strange since I have more energy and believe that I am on a path to recovery.

Saturday, September 28

Scott and I spend most of the day housecleaning. I'm not tired, and we both notice an improvement with my energy level. I feel more productive physically and mentally. We realize that we haven't done a good cleaning since early May, before my diagnosis. Afterward, Scott and I go on a long walk. I experience some mild back pain and discomfort that has been increasing through the day. I probably overdid it. I take one Advil at bedtime and sleep well. Cancer, be GONE!!!

Sunday, September 29

I wake up feeling good! My energy level continues to be better. We spend the morning doing some last-minute cleaning. The house looks great! We enjoy the rest of the day relaxing and walking in the early evening. I enjoy a good horn practice before we settle in and watch a movie.

Monday, September 30

I continue to feel noticeably better today. Something has changed. Could we be closer to complete response? My back pain is almost nonexistent, despite the increased physical activity this past weekend. Overall, my energy level has dramatically improved. I've been regular now for almost a week and my work productivity has improved due to my increased energy level. My horn practice goes well, even after skipping a couple days this week. With all the extra energy spent cleaning the house and walking, it doesn't feel like I've overexerted myself. As I practice, I continue to see a noticeable improvement. My sound is definitely stronger and better. I have more control over moving my diaphragm as I push out to support my sound. I smile as I realize this. This only reinforces my belief that my horn playing is the single best indicator for how well I'm defeating cancer. I don't need a CT scan to tell me this.

OCTOBER

....

Tuesday, October 1

It's hard to believe that it's been five months since my cancer journey began. I'm having another good day! I am regular and have little or no back pain. Sometimes it's the little things that matter. I feel as though something definitely has changed inside me. Scott and I continue to hold onto the belief that my days of cancer will soon be behind me. We're almost there!

....

Wednesday, October 2

I go into the office and work continues to go well. During my evening horn practice, my ability to take big breaths between phrasing is improving. I'm sounding better and better as I prepare for my next lesson this coming Sunday. Scott and I are leaving early Saturday afternoon to attend another Philadelphia Orchestra performance. This concert will include Rachmaninoff's Piano

Concerto no. 2 and Strauss's Alpine Symphony. We hope to connect with Jen Montone, principal horn, afterward for drinks.

§

I first met Jen, who is on faculty at Curtis Institute of Music, last
year as I was checking in for Curtis Summerfest 2018. She was in
the lobby of the hotel, having just finished a meeting. I recognized
her immediately. I felt we knew each other and went right over to
say hello. I gave her a big hug and introduced myself, in that order.
It was nice meeting and talking with Jen. It was all horn talk as
we shared some stories about our respective journeys playing the
French horn. Jen is easy to talk to. There's no pretense. She is
very positive and encouraging, not to mention uber talented, with
a beautiful horn sound. I am always inspired whenever I hear her
play. Meeting Jen Montone at my first Curtis Summerfest in 2018
was a good sign and a great way to start off my experience.

I hope she and Jack can join us on Saturday. Aside from being
a wonderful person, Jen is considered one of the world's best horn
players. She is so inspiring! Most of what Jack teaches me comes
directly from what he learns from Jen; I am very fortunate.

Thursday, October 3

As with most Thursdays, I go into the office. I feel great! I get a
little tired in the afternoon. Fortunately, I'm able to work the rest
of the day from home. Scott and I enjoy a two-mile walk before I
practice my horn. The Kopprasch Etudes that Jack assigned me
are shaping up. I think I'm in good shape for my lesson on Sunday.
I begin to take my day-before dose of dexamethasone in preparation for my seventh-cycle infusion tomorrow.

Friday, October 4

Today is my seventh infusion. Our time with Dr. CO goes very
well and is much more positive than when we first met. We are

completely aligned with the belief that I will reach complete response soon. My alkaline phosphatase is down to 216 from 242 two weeks ago. This is closer to the 150 normal range mark. Dr. CO agrees that alkaline phosphatase, although not definitive, is a prognostic indicator that the cancer is going away! All of my blood counts are returning to their normal ranges.

....

Saturday, October 5

We're off to Philly for the weekend! Jack had highly recommended hearing Strauss's Alpine symphony. It has great horn passages and is one of his favorites. There are twelve French horns plus four Wagner tubas. A Wagner tuba is a cross between a French horn and a trombone. These tubas look like euphoniums. They are played with a horn mouthpiece in the key of F or B-flat, just like a French horn. Wagner tubas were created for Richard Wagner. Wagner wrote parts for tubas in his opera cycle Der Ring des Nibelungen. Since then, Anton Bruckner and Richard Strauss also wrote parts for them in several of their works: Bruckner's 7th Symphony and Strauss's Alpine Symphony. In tonight's performance of Strauss's Alpine Symphony, there is a section at the beginning when four horn players from the orchestra actually get up out of their chairs and exit the stage through some secret panel only to be heard moments later playing a rapid rondo, a perfectly harmonized section of the symphony, off-stage that creates a horn call in the distance. The French horns are heard throughout the symphony. Jen does a superb job on the horn solos. It's super cool and sounds great!

I was able to reconnect with Jen Montone via email. I sent her a message to check in and see how she is doing. I included a You-Tube link to Jack's and my Summerfest performance of Beethoven's Sextet, op. 81b, second and third movements.

Jen sent a very kind response: *"Congrats on your Beethoven— you guys sound great together!! You're rocking it!!"* You can only imagine how much this feedback means to me!

Sunday, October 6

Scott and I sleep until 8:30 AM. This is a good thing, given that we're almost always awake by 7 AM. Although we are staying at the Westin, we head across the street to the Sofitel for breakfast. We have a delightful Sunday breakfast there. We always enjoy seeing the servers and restaurant manager, Chris.

After breakfast, I wait about an hour and then manage a partial warm-up to prepare for my horn lesson with Jack. I still feel full from eating breakfast, and the hotel room we're in has horrible acoustics. When we get to Lenfest Hall, it takes the first fifteen minutes of my lesson to complete my warm-up. Once there, I am clicking on all eight cylinders! I zip through no. 13 and no. 14 Kopprasch Etudes in Book 1 like a pro! Jack sits back in his chair listening with amazement. I like when he does this. He says this isn't the same Louis horn playing he remembers from two years ago, when we began my lessons and played together at Summerfest. He is genuinely happy for me!

Just as I think my horn lesson can't get any better, Jack pulls out the Beethoven horn excerpt that I hummed for him at the Ritz Carlton last night. Tears well up in my eyes and run down my cheeks. Jack asks what I am thinking. I can barely speak when I share that I couldn't have imagined getting to this point with my horn playing when my lung cancer journey began. But I have! I am so happy!

I sit back in my chair looking at the excerpt and then just jump in and start playing it. We then play it together and when we finish, we move on to play the horn duet from Beethoven's 8th Symphony. Aside from Summerfest, this is the first time Jack and I have played duets together since we began my horn lessons in January 2018. It sounds great! I almost can't wait to get home and practice more. Once I arrive back home, I immediately pull out my copy of Strauss's Horn Concerto no. 1 and begin practicing.

I am there! Jack says that I am "killing cancer." I am getting it out of my body. I feel it. These are the final days of cancer. Lots of smiling faces this weekend!!!

Monday, October 7

Although I wake up pain free this morning, I'm tired. Perhaps the events of the weekend caught up with me. I continue to be regular with no more constipation. I'm working from home and am having a productive day. I take a much-needed midday nap and end up resting for almost two hours. After my nap, Scott and I head out for a walk. We've been averaging about two miles a day. Fall is here, and we want to take advantage of the nice weather as long as possible. It's a cloudy day. The days will be getting darker sooner. ☹

Tuesday, October 8

I had some discomfort during the night along with some weird dreams. I wake up feeling tired. Overall I feel okay, but I have some pain on the left side at my waist area. I have a tennis elbow–type feeling on the back of my left leg. Fortunately, I'm working from home today. These types of issues are typical for the Monday and Tuesday after my Friday infusions.

Wednesday, October 9

I wake up in the middle of the night. The pain on my left side is sharper. I take an Advil and am able to go back to sleep. Later, I wake up still feeling some pain, along with fatigue and some lightheadedness, though my overall energy level is pretty good. I go into the office and am able to have a good day. As the day progresses, my pain subsides without medication. Then it shifts to my sternum. I especially feel this between phrases when I practice my horn. I believe this is my treatment working along with the physical activity involved with playing the French horn. Cancer doesn't like that. This first week after treatment has been typical as compared to previous cycles. I'm happy to have some discomfort because I believe it's telling me that my treatment is fighting the cancer and winning!

Thursday, October 10

If Monday's morning fatigue and nausea was an eight out of ten, today is a five. My left side, waist-level pain has subsided. I'm now feeling some discomfort on my right waist area. At nighttime, around 8 PM, as before, I feel a heat sensation across the lower part of my back from the left side to my right side. Scott can feel the heat coming off my skin when I ask him to check it out. This is interesting and pretty cool!

Friday, October 11

It's been a week since my seventh treatment cycle. I felt more fatigue and nausea this first week than I did the first week of my last two maintenance cycles. I hope this means that Keytruda/ Alimta is enough to eradicate the remaining cancer without carboplatin. Scott and I are up to walking three miles a day now.

Saturday, October 12

I wake up feeling great! Scott and I spent the day running errands. I have plenty of energy. It is a perfect fall day: cool, in the low 70s, light breeze and sunny. We walk 3.5 miles and spend the time catching up on our work week, sharing stories. I'm happy to breathe deeper and control my air flow better while playing my horn.

Sunday, October 13

It's been a good weekend. Scott and I went to Green Park, which is north on the Perkiomen Trail. We walked over three miles. There is a small lake in the park that we walked around and followed the trail back to where we parked. Along the way, we saw a woman riding a horse. The horse was beautiful and very graceful. Since my journey began, I find myself reflecting on memories of my childhood. I'm not sure why, but at that moment I thought back to when I was about eleven years old and my older brother was cast as the Fiddler in a production of *Fiddler on the Roof*. The summer play series was sponsored by the City of Scranton, and the show was performed in an open trailer with an extended stage in parks throughout the city. I remember that day well. It was the day I had my first doctor's appointment, or at least the first doctor's appointment I can remember going to on my own. I remember how thin I was: 119 pounds. I was slightly malnourished and anemic. This didn't surprise me, since my mom had four of us to feed all on her own. These types of events define us as we grow up. It's amazing what we remember from our past. I like when Scott and I share stories as we walk.

Monday, October 14

I continue to have discomfort in my left lower back near my waist. It's annoying as it comes and goes, but I keep smiling and continue to power through. I slept well and have more energy this week as compared to last. This is my second week post seventh cycle. I know by now that anything can happen this week. It can be a good week or one full of surprises. Either way, I remain hopeful that a complete response is near.

Tuesday, October 15

I'm still experiencing some nausea and fatigue as the day progresses. I take half a tablet, 5 mg, of Compazine, and it seems to work right away. I've been taking half a tablet of Compazine on and off before bedtime for nausea. My discomfort and pain are moderate and seem to shift from the left to the right side of my lower waist area. My right latissimus has been bothersome as well. I'm not sure if this is from walking more or from the cancer or both. Because of this, I take the day off from practicing my horn. Scott and I enjoy our daily walk.

Wednesday, October 16

Today is a better day. I reflect on the ups and downs of my days and am reminded how unpredictable cancer can be. I'm happy to have a very productive day at the office. My horn practice this evening isn't ideal. Sometimes I have a challenging rehearsal after taking a day off. It's important to keep my embouchure conditioned so that the muscles stay strong. I relax and end up having a good practice session.

Thursday, October 17

I wake up feeling great! I haven't felt like this in a while. I have more energy, with no fatigue or nausea. I travel to our Kenilworth, New Jersey, office for a lunch meeting with our vice president of lung marketing, Piero. Our lunch meeting goes well. Piero might be adding a new position on his global lung marketing team. I share my interest. We talked about my background in lung cancer along with my own personal journey.

I end up walking two miles today, and my horn practice session is back on track!

Friday, October 18

I wake up around 1 AM with nausea and pain. I take half a Compazine and an Advil. I'm able to go back to sleep around 2 AM until 7:45 AM. Mild fatigue returns and although I continue to have nausea throughout the day, all goes well with my workday.

Saturday, October 19

I feel good today. My horn rehearsal goes well, just in time for my lesson tomorrow. Scott and I are headed back to Philly to attend a Philadelphia Orchestra concert of Mahler's 5th Symphony tonight, and then I'll have my horn lesson with Jack tomorrow morning.

Sunday, October 20

The concert last night was fantastic! Jen's "Corno Obligato" solo in Mahler's 5th (third movement, the scherzo) was uber amazing! Scott and I were able to meet Jen at Volvér, a restaurant attached to the Kimmel Center, at a reception following the concert. It was great seeing her again. Before she left, we walked with her out into the Kimmel Center hallway where we were alone. I shared with her the news of my lung cancer. It was a somber moment. Jen was immediately concerned and very supportive. She sent me an inspiring email the following week that I hold dearly to my heart.

Scott and I enjoy breakfast this morning and a break before I have to warm up for my horn lesson at noon. Although I'm not able to complete my full warm-up, I have a good lesson anyway. It rains all day. Scott and I spend the rest of the day relaxing and enjoy a midday nap together. I experience some pain and discomfort in my left pelvis area that wraps around to my left side back area near the waist. It seems to originate in my back, in the vicinity of my left lower lung lobe where my primary tumor is.

The pain shoots down my left leg to the calf. I feel my knee pulse like tennis elbow. It isn't too bad, just annoying. Scott and I cuddle on the family room sofa while watching a movie. I feel safe, and if for only that moment, that everything is going to be okay and someday I'll be cancer free. I smile inside as I know this pain is just another pathetic attempt by the cancer to discourage me. I believe the cancer is making some last-ditch effort to survive. Good luck with that, because I know that my cancer is on its way out!

Monday, October 21

My pain and discomfort have subsided, as it always has. I'm happy to be working from home today. It's a productive day. As usual, I have some fatigue later in the afternoon and take a short nap. It's been three weeks since my seventh treatment cycle, the third maintenance cycle of Keytruda/Alimta. So far, I feel better in comparison to the same time with previous cycles. I'm feeling stronger despite the pain and fatigue. My episodes of pain and discomfort are fewer and less eventful, and their durations are shorter. These are all good signs that I'm crushing the cancer!

Tuesday, October 22

I feel similar to how I felt yesterday. Pain and discomfort are a three out of ten. My eighth cycle (fourth maintenance cycle) of Keytruda and Alimta is scheduled for this coming Friday. I feel good going into this next treatment cycle.

I have been invited to be a guest speaker at a Merck Global Oncology Medical Affairs (GOMA) annual meeting tomorrow in Princeton, New Jersey. They arranged to have a driver bring me directly from home to the meeting and back. This eliminates the stress of driving myself. The attendees will be Merck's Global medical teams of physicians, pharmacy directors and clinical support personnel. An estimated three hundred or more people will be in the audience. All are Merck director level or above. This will be the second time I've shared my lung cancer journey with my colleagues at Merck. As mentioned, the first time was at the end of August, at the off-site conference center, in front of a group of 150 newly hired oncology sales representatives. I am excited and happy to receive another opportunity, though it continues to be a bit surreal to be talking about me having lung cancer. It feels different when you say it out loud. I know I will see my Global associates, some of whom know that someone from Merck will be sharing their lung cancer journey, but they most likely will not know it's me until they see me on stage.

I spent my first two years at Merck in Learning and Development, prior to my current position in Biomarker Promotions. In Biomarker Promotions I had Global, in addition to U.S. responsibilities up until a few months ago when a new employee was hired to take over the Global Biomarker side. Creating this new position makes sense given our rapid Global growth. I know my colleagues will see me and think I'm facilitating the patient journey portion, not realizing right away that I am the patient. Surely this will be eye-opening for them and for me when I voice the reality of my own situation, out loud, in front of my friends and Global colleagues. I must admit, I'm a bit apprehensive and nervous about this. But I am committed to helping others, first and foremost, so I'll set my own apprehension aside for now and power through this moment with my larger goal in mind. My journey will provide valuable insights from the patient's point of view. This is what we do—all of us who support Keytruda at Merck. I am committed to offering whatever insights and information I can to help shape this effort. This makes me happy and proud.

....

Wednesday, October 23

I have a good night's sleep and wake up excited about my speaking engagement today. I'm focused on the positive aspects of what my purpose is and what I want to communicate to my colleagues. My friend and colleague, Dr. Linda, will be on stage with me to facilitate our discussion. I arrive at the Princeton Westin about ninety minutes before our segment. I wanted to arrive early so I could acclimate to the environment. I try to settle in and think about what key points I want to share and how I want to say them, but I continue to think this is surreal. Dr. Linda will walk through the questions and shape the discussion. I like this. She facilitated our talk in August, with the 150 newly hired oncology sales representatives, so I am very comfortable with her style. We've developed a good relationship. I trust Dr. Linda. She's very supportive.

We meet outside the ballroom and walk in together. I see the size of the room and immediately feel very overwhelmed. It hits me what I'll be doing. The magnitude of how large the room is with a few hundred attendees—I wonder if I can do this. Dr. Linda picks up on my hesitation and offers to take me on stage to settle in and get accustomed to the view from the stage so that I can be more comfortable.

In the hallway I see Piero, with whom I had lunch just last week. It's good to see a friendly, familiar face before I go on stage. Back in the ballroom, Dr. Linda introduces me to the senior executives who lead this global medical group. They are genuine and very welcoming. One in particular is a senior vice president, and a physician, who is the head of this group, based in the U.K. He is welcoming and very kind. Then I meet the U.S. vice president, who is also a physician. She is very supportive. I thank them both for the honor of being invited to share my journey.

We were given forty-five minutes for our discussion, but the previous presenters went over on their time. Based on this, Dr. Linda and I make the decision to condense our discussion to thirty minutes; fortunately, this ends up being enough time. The talk goes well. I tailor my presentation to what a medical group would be interested in hearing. I am passionate on behalf of the patient and, I think, engaging.

I am open, honest and very candid about my journey. Perhaps almost too candid. At times I get tearful as I relive the moment I found out I had cancer. I hold the tears back as best I can when I tell the story of going to the doctor for what I believed was a herniated disc in my back only to be told I had lesions on my spine. This is the moment that changed my life forever. I wonder how my colleagues feel hearing this. I keep speaking, still feeling this is all surreal. It's hard to believe that my journey began just five months ago and even harder to believe it's "me" here living with stage 4, metastatic non-small cell lung cancer.

So many emotions go through my head as I present, but I manage to stay on track. Above all, and however my journey plays out, I am committed to helping all lung cancer patients, however I can, through my own experiences.

I feel good at the end of our discussion. I believe that I was able to communicate my journey effectively to the audience. Working at Merck, supporting Keytruda, means the world to me. I repeat: there is no such thing as a coincidence.

Several colleagues come up to me afterward to offer their support. They share their amazement with my journey, having just found out about my lung cancer. Everyone is great. We hug and take a few selfies together. A colleague I have not met before from Finland comes up to me. She shares a story of a friend who is going through a similar situation and is very complimentary on my presentation. She politely asks for a picture and permission to share on their internal blog. I agree and am honored to be asked. What a wonderful experience! Could inspirational speaking be my future?

....

Thursday, October 24

I'm back in the office today with 224 emails to catch up on after being out for one day. Yikes! Fortunately, I don't have many conference calls, so I am able to catch up with few interruptions.

Shortly after 10 AM, I take my first dose of dexamethasone in preparation for my eighth treatment infusion tomorrow. I only need to take half a pill since carboplatin is no longer part of my treatment. Overall, my maintenance treatment is much more tolerable than when I was on the triplet of Alimta, carboplatin and Keytruda.

Nausea returns today so I take half a Compazine tablet at night and end up taking the other half just before going to sleep.

Friday, October 25

I wake up early to get ready for my treatment appointment. My good friend Lisa will be coming by at 7:45 AM to pick me up. I laugh to myself when I notice the forgotten Ambien tablet on my nightstand. Oh, well, I'll look forward to a nap later in the day, after my infusion, and not make that mistake again tonight when I go to bed.

I'm so happy that Lisa will be with me. Scott is away in Tampa on an important business trip. He left Tuesday night and will be away through next Wednesday. Lisa graciously offered to stand in for Scott during my infusion at the cancer center.

Lisa arrives right on time and we enjoy coffee from our Jura machine. She loves coffee from our Swiss coffee maker. We leave for the cancer center and arrive on time. I introduce Lisa to Dr. CO. The appointment goes well. The doctor continues to react positively to information I share on how I'm feeling since my last infusion, and is pleased with how I look and feel. My weight continues to be very consistent, still holding at 170 pounds. I ask Dr. CO to review my baseline May 15 CT scan against the latest August 19 CT scan with Lisa. Dr. CO points out the areas where the cancer has shrunk or is gone and confirms the date for my next CT scan, Monday morning, November 11, at the Blue Bell Radiology Center. Lisa and I proceed to the infusion suite to begin my eighth cycle. Blood is drawn. It turns out that my platelets are elevated due to dehydration. I consciously have been drinking more water since my journey started, but I must admit I have forgotten to drink enough this past week. Not sure how that happened. In order to ensure that I am hydrated properly prior to receiving my treatment, the nurse infuses saline. I'm able to have this infused while simultaneously receiving my treatment infusion medications. All goes well during my treatment, and Lisa and I are on our way home when Dr. CO calls. My alkaline phosphatase actually went up a little, versus continuing to go down. It is 258 versus 216 the previous time, prior to the seventh cycle. I am concerned that it's gone up and wonder what might be going on. Dr. CO says not to be. If it were 700 there would be concern, but 258 is essentially flat as compared to last time. Dr. CO says my overall blood work shows improvement to normal ranges, in particular my red blood cell count, which has been low. My thyroid-stimulating hormone (TSH) continues to be in the normal range, but the number is now 96 versus 46 last time. This is a stronger "normal" number.

On our way home, I treat Lisa to lunch at Basta Pasta in Skippack. I really enjoyed our day together! I always like learning more about Lisa whenever we're together. We've become close friends since my first Curtis Summerfest performance in 2018. Lisa has been there every step of the way since my cancer journey began.

I immediately take a nap when I get home. During my nap, I begin to feel some pain and discomfort in that same lower left side of my back. It increases, so I'm only able to rest for thirty minutes despite how tired I am. Scott and I are able to connect before I go for a walk. My strength is good during my walk. I really don't experience any discomfort or pain. I walk two miles and practice my horn afterward. The pain returns during practice, but I power through and end up having a good session. Afterward I have difficulty trying to get comfortable sitting down watching TV. I consistently find myself shifting from my left side to my right. I try lying down, but that doesn't help. I am very uncomfortable and don't understand why. The pain is increasing. I'm really getting pissed off now. I begin swearing! This helps me feel better. I resort to a Diclofenac Epolamine pain patch. It helps, but I still am unable to get comfortable. This is the first time I've had pain right after an infusion. Could this be that Keytruda/Alimta are doing their thing? Kill that damn cancer already!

I go into the bedroom and watch TV from bed. This helps. I take an Advil, which I haven't had to take in quite some time. The pain immediately begins to dissipate. It's only 8:30 PM, so I binge-watch several episodes of *Big Bang Theory*. I love this series because it makes me laugh! I continue swearing and laughing, waiting for the pain to pass, knowing this is another pathetic attempt for the cancer to try to discourage me. I wake up at 2 AM to go to the bathroom and feel better, as if it never happened.

Saturday, October 26

Yep, it's the middle of the night, and I'm pain free as I head to the bathroom. I see a text from Scott with a time of 3:32 AM. He was still working! He had a product release or what Scott refers to as a "Go Live" meeting with his client. It was global launch on a new cloud solution, so it was all hands on deck throughout the night to ensure the execution of the new solution was successful. Scott calls me at 7:30 AM to see how I am doing. I am more concerned about his lack of sleep. He only had four hours of sleep last night.

I always enjoy talking with Scott. He has a very calming voice and is always positive. This morning I'm scared about what's going on with my pain. I haven't felt this bad since I was first diagnosed. Scott and I plan on reconnecting later in the day to see how I'm doing. Our fingers are crossed. I run some errands and practice my horn. So far, so good; no pain today.

It's been a while since our dear friend Alisha and I have connected. I sent her a text last week with hopes of connecting sometime this weekend, though I'm not one to dump my stuff on friends. Scott and I have always relied on each other for support and rarely reach out to anyone else.

Scott and I reconnect in the afternoon. He is happy that I'm feeling better. We discuss our plans for our Celebration of Life, Love and Friendship planned for mid-November. We're happy to be doing this for all our dear friends and coworkers at Merck who have supported us throughout my journey. I enjoy a good horn rehearsal. It's nice day, partly cloudy and cool. I can't wait until Scott comes home.

....

Sunday, October 27

I wake up feeling good this morning. I had my day-after dose of dexamethasone yesterday. The dexamethasone seems to wear off during the middle of the day, as I began feeling tired with some discomfort and pain returning in the lower left area of my back, the same area my pain mostly occurs. So far, my fatigue isn't as bad now while I'm on Alimta/Keytruda as it was during my first four cycles of Keytruda Combo. Carboplatin is the strongest of the three Combo agents, so it makes sense to have less fatigue without it. This is a very good thing since barring any disease progression, this will most likely be my treatment every three weeks for the next two years. This treatment aligns with the Keynote-189 clinical study for Keytruda Combo.

The one thing I realized most these past three days is how much I rely on Scott. He's been so incredible all through my journey. He is extremely patient and very kind, always. He does so many little things that help so much. Most of all, it's how he does them, lovingly. He looks at me when I'm in pain, and I can see in his eyes that he wishes he could take all my pain away in a heartbeat.

This Sunday is not very good in comparison to other post-treatment Sundays. It feels like the cancer is still there fighting, resisting being terminated. Today I feel like I'm crawling to the finish line. I decide not to practice my horn today. I'm not feeling well enough. I go into our bedroom early to lie down and watch TV. I feel more comfortable lying down. I end up falling asleep early. I remember dreaming about my wonderful dalmatian, Tiffany. She was the light of my life, the best dog ever!

Scott comes home on Wednesday. I'm counting the days.

Monday, October 28

Monday seems to be starting just like Sunday ended. I am in pain and discomfort with some nausea. This isn't a good combination. I work from home and power through the day. A mid-afternoon nap helps. I return to practicing my horn despite how I feel. I actually have a good practice today! My sound continues to be strong and controlled. I begin working on the Strauss Horn Concerto no. 1. I haven't played this piece since 1985. It's a very energetic and regal piece for the French horn. I smile as I reflect on my college days when I played this fearlessly.

§

I have another memory of home from further back, when I was about eight years old. It was right before the holidays. Our family Christmas tree was up. You know the kind that was all silver with classic ornaments that came with a slowly rotating light changer on the floor positioned so the tree seemed to change colors from red, to blue, to green and then to back to gold—a classic 1960s tree. I was in the kitchen, on the floor, near the baseboard radiator where it was warm; it was cold outside with a lot of snow on the ground. Mom was cooking dinner for us as I sat cutting out paper snowflakes, using Elmer's glue to add red and green glitter. I remember how I felt in that moment: safe, content and loved. I remember how happy I was. This is one of my happiest childhood memories.

Tuesday, October 29

Scott calls this morning, as he always does when he travels. I call it my *good morning, wake-up call!* He shares that he is starting a new account and will need to travel (again) for a three-day trip to Raleigh, North Carolina, on November 17. This is the day after our Life, Love and Friendship celebration. The timing for this news couldn't be any worse. I am so upset with the timing of this trip, especially since it has been such a challenging week with him not here. I am so upset that I immediately shut down and get quiet. This is never good.

Wednesday, October 30

I went to bed last night without talking to Scott. I can't remember ever doing this. I was so upset that my heart ached. Scott and I never fight, but I was so hurt by this news that I didn't know what to do, so my immediate go-to place was to shut down. Today I wake up still very upset from Scott telling me about his next business trip. I am hurt and disappointed that he will be leaving the day after our Celebration event. I have a voicemail from Scott waiting for me when I wake up. He is concerned that he hasn't heard from me in over twenty-four hours. I feel so bad, but I can't bring myself to talk about it. I am feeling the emotional impact of my withdrawing. As a diversion, I go into the office. I am so upset that I end up crying at my desk. A few coworkers notice and offer solace. Although I'm embarrassed, their support means the world to me.

I go into a privacy room to call Scott and do my best to share how I feel without attacking him. We have a good talk. Of course, I cry. I love him so much. I wish none of this was happening. As always, his voice calms me. We agree to continue our conversation tonight when he returns home.

I take a nap when I get home from work. Naps always help, but I feel the same as I did yesterday, sore and nauseous. This first week after my eighth cycle seems so much different from any other first-week cycle. I'm not sure what's going on. I'm scared. I remind myself that this truly is a journey. I've had so many ups and downs, twist and turns since this all started. This is just another unexpected twist to add to the list. I'll be ok. Cancer didn't happen overnight, and it's not going to go away overnight. I'm just impatient and want it gone now!

Scott gets home at 9 PM. I am literally in bed moaning with pain. We have a heartfelt talk and decide that any business trips, moving forward, will be limited to three days until I reach complete response. I cry as we talk. I'm a pretty strong person but for the first time since my journey began, the emotional component of what we are going through is impacting us like nothing else before.

Thursday, October 31

Happy Halloween! I'm feeling better today but continue to experience pain, discomfort and some nausea. Perhaps feeling a little better is due to Scott being home. I'll take it. I go into the office for meetings, and surprisingly I'm able to get through the day. Despite how I'm feeling this week, Scott and I keep up our walks. I have a good practice session this evening as I prepare for my next horn lesson with Jack. I'm so happy that Scott is home. I know in my heart that together we can meet any challenge.

NOVEMBER

Friday, November 1

I'm feeling similar to how I've felt this past week. I was really hoping to be feeling better in time for Victoria and Steve's wedding tomorrow. Victoria is a work colleague. I recommended her to my previous manager as a candidate to fill my vacant position in oncology learning and development when I moved to my Biomarker Promotions role.

I work from home and enjoy a nice nap at the end of the day. I'm feeling nauseous and decide not to practice tonight. Instead, Scott and I review our to do list for our Celebration event in two weeks.

Saturday, November 2

Victoria's and Steve's wedding is beautiful! Victoria is a stunning bride. We meet Sharon and Hank, Victoria's mom and dad, along with Bob, Steve's dad, and his girlfriend Frances. We are seated at the same table as Kaye and Mark, Victoria's sister and brother-in-law. We enjoy our time with them. The ceremony is perfect, and the DJ music is from the '70s. The beat is good throughout the night.

The night is vibrant as everyone celebrates. I find myself very uncomfortable sitting in my chair. My back is really bothering me. I am able to find a sofa on the lower level of the building where Scott and I hang out for a while. Unfortunately, the sofa is away from the wedding festivities, so we soon return to join the dance crowd upstairs. Scott has a great time dancing! No dancing for me tonight due to my back pain. I hang in there until 9 PM, when my pain becomes too much to tolerate. Nonetheless, we had a great time. I'm so glad I was able to be there. It was a beautiful wedding!

Sunday, November 3

I had another good night's sleep last night. That's two in a row—yeah! I have a good warm-up mid-morning before heading to Philadelphia for my lesson. Once again Jack shows amazement with my horn playing! He points out how strong I sound and how my breathing has improved. I know my horn sound is so much stronger than it was in mid-August when I had my last CT scan. Jack's reaction reinforces my belief that I don't need a CT scan to tell me that I'm getting better. My horn playing is the best indicator of how my lungs are doing.

....

Monday, November 4

It's Katie Couric day! Katie has been a big cancer advocate since her husband, Jay Monahan, was just age forty-two when he died of colon cancer in 1998. Scott and I have been invited to a Patient Journey Forum organized by Merck's senior vice president, Jill. Katie Couric is the moderator. It's Keytruda's five-year anniversary. There are four patients; two have metastatic melanoma, one has metastatic non-small cell lung cancer; and one has metastatic Lynch Syndrome, MSI-H.[32] They were part of our Keynote-001 clinical trial (Merck's first Keytruda clinical trial). These four patients paved the way for all other patients, including myself. Through their treatment, Merck medical teams were able to capture patient-level clinical data that has helped Merck determine the path forward for Keytruda across all tumor types. All four patients seemed to be at death's doorstep when they began treatment with Keytruda. Their experiences are truly inspirational and reinforce my own hope for survival. At the end of the session, Scott and I receive the opportunity to

----

[32] Lynch syndrome (LS) is an adult-onset, cancer predisposition syndrome. It is caused by a mutation in one of the genes involved in the mismatch repair (MMR) pathway. Individuals with LS are at increased risk for colon and other cancers, including gastric, urinary tract, brain, small bowel, pancreatic, hepatobiliary and sebaceous carcinoma. Screening tests and genetic testing are used to diagnose Lynch syndrome. One test looks for changes that indicate the gene that affects DNA repairs is not working. These changes are called microsatellite instability or MSI. Tumors that have microsatellite instability are called MSI-high (MSI-H). *Source:* The Jackson Laboratory: *https://www.jax.org/education-and-learning/ clinical-and-continuing-education/cancer-resources/lynch-syndrome*

meet Katie and get a photograph together. During this time, I am able to share my diagnosis with her. Katie is authentic and genuinely expresses concern for me. I'm so glad that we were able to meet her.

As we return home, I am really tired. The morning events have taken an emotional toll on me. I take a nap and, as always, feel better afterward. Scott and I enjoy a nice dinner. After a break, I practice and have a good session. I'm really making progress on the Strauss Horn Concerto no. 1.

....

Tuesday, November 5

I wake up feeling rested but with pain in my left pelvic area. The pain is sharp and annoying: about a six out of ten. Despite this, I go into the office. Afterward, Scott and I go for our walk without me feeling any additional discomfort. I'm able to maintain a good energy level throughout the day.

....

Wednesday, November 6

I wake up with sharp pain now on the left side of my waist in the pelvic area. I had two episodes of interrupted sleep, around 1 AM and again at 4 AM, from pain and discomfort. I go into the office and power through my workday. I'm still not sure what's going on. Days of feeling good are followed by more days of feeling bad, with pain, discomfort and nausea. I feel like there's a battle going on with the cancer inside my body. My skin is hot to the touch. I've experienced this before. I hope it means Keytruda/Alimta is burning the cancer away. I have several meetings throughout my workday and end up having to take an Advil during the day just before noontime. This is unusual, since I haven't taken anything for pain midday in a while. One of my meetings is with my coworker and friend Mitch. We've worked together since I started at Merck. Mitch is a good friend. He genuinely cares and supports my journey. It's always good to see a friendly face when you're not feeling well.

I take a nap immediately after getting home. This helps, but my pelvic pain continues. I end up having to take another Advil at bedtime. My pain is about a six on a pain scale, just enough to be annoying. I end up having a good night of uninterrupted sleep anyway.

Thursday, November 7

I get up feeling okay, but the pain soon reappears as my day progresses. I decide to work from home to avoid overexerting myself. The pain continues to radiate from the left side of my pelvic area. Aside from this, my nausea is better and there's no pain or discomfort anywhere else in my body. Scott and I begin cleaning the house for the big Celebration of Life, Love and Friendship next Saturday. There's a lot to do. We decided to put the stake in the ground and thank everyone, our friends, including our Merck family, for all their love and support over the past six months. Our goal was to have a complete response by now. We were hoping that I would be cancer free in time for our Celebration event. Either way, this day is going to be about our celebration with our friends, not cancer.

Except for today, I went into the office every day this week. Tomorrow I have an important meeting so I'll be going back in.

My pain is worse between 5 PM and bedtime. I find myself taking Advil each night before I go to bed. This makes me comfortable so I can fall asleep. It's like clockwork. In the middle of the night at about 2 AM, the pain is gone. Maybe this cycle of pain followed by no pain is due to physical activity: going into the office and walking two miles per day. I really don't know. As I reflect on the pain that I've been experiencing, I realize that right about at the third week of my seventh cycle—my third treatment of Keytruda/Alimta maintenance cycle—approximately one month ago, is when my regular pain and discomfort started. Something is definitely going on.

....

Friday, November 8

The pain in the left pelvic area continues. I feel it in my sternum as well. Scott and I continue to wonder why I'm experiencing pain. We thought I would be pain-free by this time given that I am far into my Keytruda maintenance treatment program. Especially since I had such a good response back in early summer when my treatment began. I keep working and powering through the pain. I go into the office today as planned. This is my fourth day in the office this week. I know that it may sound crazy—"why am I working right now?"—but working for me is a positive distraction. This is not how I planned on ending my career so I will continue to work as long as possible. I believe that I'll know when it's time to unplug from working. Until then, I am committed to getting back to a normal work schedule.

....

Saturday, November 9

Scott and I spend most of the morning cleaning the house to prepare for our party. I make time to practice my horn so as not to miss a day. At noon, Scott and I leave for State College to see our friend Eryn. We're planning on staying the night since it's about a three-hour drive. This will give us more time with Eryn. We didn't get to see her much while visiting Cherie and Dean in Zug.

Eryn is very smart, independent and tough. Despite her dad receiving a Global marketing position that brought them to move to Switzerland, Eryn is committed to finishing college at Penn State main campus in State College, Pennsylvania. Given how far she is from her family, Scott and I have become her surrogate uncles. We love Eryn and her family and are happy to be there for support anytime. We enjoy the drive to State College. It's cold outside, around

40°F. On the way, Tchaikovsky's 6th Symphony, "Pathétique," is on the radio. This is such a sad symphony, especially the last movement. It's the last symphony Tchaikovsky wrote. He died shortly after he finished composing it. Tchaikovsky struggled with his homosexuality. His 4th Symphony speaks to "destiny." I always feel like he's crying as he writes the last movement of his 6th Symphony. It's like he knows it's his last symphony and he's saying goodbye. Perhaps true to who he was, Tchaikovsky had something defining planned for his last symphony. He led the first performance in Saint Petersburg on October 28, 1893, nine days before his death.[33]

[33.] *Music:* Tchaikovsky Symphony no. 6 in B Minor, op. 74, "Pathétique." Eugene Ormandy and the Philadelphia Orchestra (YouTube video, 46:38). Please go to minute 44:36 to hear the dramatic ending. Posted by cgoroo, September 30, 2017; accessed September 2020. *https://www.youtube.com/watch?v=mGz8vJeVI8Y*

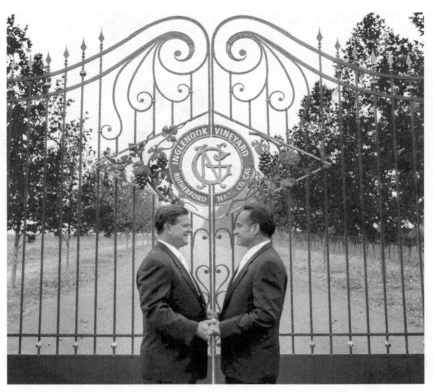

At the front gate of the Inglenook winery at our 25ᵗʰ Anniversary Celebration event, November 2018

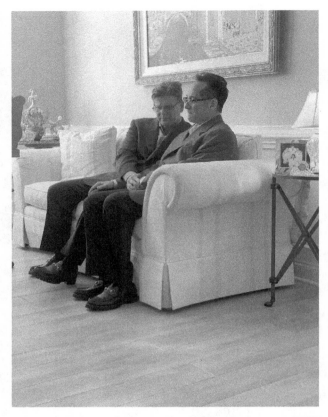

Listening to the Prelude and Fugue No. 1 in C major, BWV 846 from the Well-Tempered Clavier at our Celebration of Life, Love and Friendship Event, November 2019

Part III
Courage

Movement 3
Adagio molto e cantabile[34]

This movement is much slower than the others. Each *note moves with deliberation. In music technical language, "cantabile" refers to an instrumental piece that, in some way, might easily be sung by a human voice. For example, "adagio molto cantabile" means the piece should be played slowly and sweetly as a song.*

[34.] *Music:* Beethoven Symphony no. 9 in D Minor, op. 125 "Choral." The Mormon Tabernacle Choir, Eugene Ormandy and the Philadelphia Orchestra (YouTube video, 1:08:14). Minute 29:06 marks the beginning of the third movement. Posted by soy ink, August 24, 2017; accessed September 2020. *https://www.youtube.com/watch?v=eb_vUFxgtxM*

My heart and soul are moved as I listen to this movement. It seems sad yet hopeful and perfectly depicts this part of my journey. For me, having courage means digging deep within myself to find the strength to move forward under the worst of conditions. Fighting stage 4 lung cancer is the biggest challenge I've had. Nothing in my experience can compare. Like many of us, I work hard to maintain my positive attitude.

Courage permits us to manage our fear as we face extreme dangers and difficulties. When I look back and think about things I've been afraid of in the past, I remind myself to remember how it feels to be on the other side of that equation. How will I feel afterward if I meet this latest challenge head-on? Asking this question gives me the strength to dig deep to figure it out. What's the alternative? Succumbing to the challenge isn't an option I choose to allow myself. It's okay to be afraid, because spirit and bravery can overcome any fear. I believe the feeling of overcoming a challenge outweighs the fear of that challenge.

Personal integrity has been my guide throughout my life. Sometimes I think of myself as a superhero, hence my self-given moniker Louis 2.0. Thinking outside myself this way helps me cope with cancer. Having a sense of humor doesn't hurt, either. I've found myself laughing in the face of cancer many times through my journey. Cancer doesn't even come close to defining who I am. It is nothing more than a speed bump in life. Speed bumps can be removed and eliminated. They are a mere distraction. Living life is more important to me than living in fear. This is my truth.

I shared that this movement of Beethoven's Symphony no. 9 in D Minor seems sad. Sad in that we sometimes forget how much power we have over our destiny. It reminds me of all that's good. All that I believe I can be. I intuit this may have been what Beethoven was thinking when he wrote this movement. It is reflective of what was, what might have been and hope for what may come.

November

....

Monday, November 11

I have another CT scan today. By all accounts, today's scan should support a complete response based on the trajectory that has been established since I started treatment. After the first two Keytruda Combo cycles, my July CT scan showed a 50 percent reduction in cancer, and after two more Keytruda Combo cycles, my August CT scan showed an 80 percent reduction in cancer. So, there is an expectation, based on this information, that we should be closer to or at the finish line with this latest CT scan.

The CT scan goes well in the morning, though the IV needle hurts upon injection and leaves a bad black and blue mark when it is taken out. This isn't a pleasant experience. I work from home the rest of the day.

....

Tuesday, November 12

I'm happy to have this latest CT scan completed. Now comes the waiting. Scott and I are definitely more anxious this time to hear the results given all the good news since August's scan. Typically, it takes two days to receive the results, so I'm looking to hear from my community oncologist by end-of-day Wednesday. We know something is different this time, as I am experiencing more pain and fatigue similar to how I felt at the beginning of my treatment at the end of May. Today I have about 60 percent energy level. I decide to work from home, just to play it safe. I am planning on going into the office tomorrow for a ninety-minute meeting starting at 3:30 PM. I'm doing a presentation on biomarkers, and then I'll be sharing my lung cancer journey with my promotional marketing colleagues. I'm really feeling fatigue and my pain is about a seven. I wish I felt better. I am scared as to why I don't. I can't wait until I get my CT scan results.

Wednesday, November 13

I wake up feeling very fatigued with continued pain, so I decide that it's best to work from home until I have to leave for my 3:30 PM presentations. I continue to be very anxious as I wait for my CT scan results. The timing of this scan strangely coincides with our Celebration of Life, Love and Friendship event this Saturday. I'm so glad I made the decision to work from home part of the day. Normally, I power through my workday when I feel this way, but knowing how much of an emotional drain I will be experiencing, working from home is best.

As part of our monthly promotional marketing staff meeting, with the support of my current manager, I create a "Biomarker: Weaving the Story" PowerPoint presentation. In my presentation I will walk through how biomarkers in oncology have evolved through the years. As a real-world example, I will also share my lung cancer journey. My "Biomarker: Weaving the Story" presentation will take the first thirty minutes, and my lung cancer journey's story will follow for the next thirty minutes. Our meeting will end with a question-and-answer session. The promotional leadership team has dubbed this monthly staff meeting as Louis Day!

By sharing my journey, my hope is to provide valuable cancer patient insights that will help my colleagues better understand what patients go through. We've all been supporting Keytruda over the past five years, and sometimes we tend to lose focus on the patient as we work hard to prepare and execute all the various cancer indications for Keytruda. Just before I begin my first biomarker presentation, I share with the group that I'm waiting for an important call from my community oncologist regarding CT scan results. Hearing this, my colleagues become as anxious as I am to hear the news. A call comes in at 4 PM that ends up going directly to voicemail, but it is not the call from the doctor. It is completely unrelated.

I'm happy to get through both presentations. At the end of my Journey presentation, my colleagues are quiet. I don't know what to think. The silence seems almost deafening, as if everyone has gasped hearing the real-world experience of a lung cancer patient. I can only imagine what it is like for them to hear a coworker, someone they've known for years, share their journey with lung cancer. I think that the details of my journey hit them hard. After a few moments that seem to last forever, everyone claps. For me, it is a somber moment as surreal turns into reality. Everyone is very kind and extremely supportive.

After the meeting, I am in a fog as I walk to my car. I am stiffer from the pain, and more tired and emotionally exhausted than I've ever felt in the past after sharing my journey. With no call yet, I wonder when I will receive the update on my scan. About a mile from the office, as I make my way home, I finally receive the call about my CT results. I can tell from Dr. CO's voice that it isn't good news. I'm upset and immediately pull over and stop the car. The cancer is growing. It's back in areas where it had disappeared. The primary tumor has grown to 3 × 3 cm, which is almost exactly where it was when it was first identified in the CT scan in May. I'm totally blown away to hear that the reality of what I've been experiencing over the past two months was not the cancer going away, but coming back. I manage to hold back the tears as I listen to Dr. CO's assessment. I am stunned. How could I have missed this? It looks like my positivity kept me from considering all possibilities. It all makes sense now as I start thinking about the symptoms I've been experiencing since the third week of my seventh cycle and throughout the past three weeks of my eighth cycle. The cancer overall is still about 60 percent gone, but we've lost some ground. This accounts for the pain and fatigue I've been experiencing. How am I going to tell Scott? With this news of my disease progression, it looks like I'll be moving on to our Plan B: Tagrisso. For my infusion treatment scheduled for Friday, Dr. CO recommends moving forward with only Alimta. There needs to be a washout period of three to six weeks from the last dose of Keytruda until the time the treatment with the tyrosine kinase inhibitor Tagrisso begins, otherwise there could be some adverse reactions if we start the TKI/EGFR too soon.

This latest CT scan was for my primary tumor only. I immediately wonder what's going on in my brain and spine. I discuss this with Dr. CO and they agree. We schedule MRIs for both my brain and spine on Wednesday, November 27, right before Thanksgiving.

After the call, I have a haircut appointment. I am meeting Scott there. This is not the time or place to share this kind of news. Scott is in the chair getting his haircut when I arrive. I don't want to tell him while we're out in public. Because of the doctor's call, I was late getting there. I can't look Scott in the eye when he asks if I've heard from Dr. CO yet regarding my CT scan results. I lie and say no as I look away to avoid crying right there in the hair salon. I've never lied to Scott, ever. The fact that I've done so now makes me even more upset. I am dazed as I get my haircut. A million thoughts run through my mind, with the number one question being: how much time do I have left? I'm ready to burst into tears by the time we get home. As soon as we walk in the door, I tell Scott the news as tears stream down my cheeks. The look on his face, and in his eyes, is not something I'll ever forget.

§

In 2013, we celebrated Scott's fiftieth birthday in Salzburg, Austria, and Venice, Italy. We began our trip in Salzburg, where we attended the Salzburg Festival. That may sound familiar because it is right out of *The Sound of Music*. Near the end of the movie, the Trapp Family Singers perform in the Salzburg Festival. The festival actually does occur every year, in July and August. How cool is that! Since we were staying in a castle just outside the city, we hired a driver to take us to an opera performance of Richard Wagner's *Die Meistersinger von Nürnberg*. The driver arrived in a black

1957 Rolls Royce limousine, very sharp and very classy. Scott and I felt like movie stars as we drove through Old Town Salzburg.

I hired a photographer to take pictures in the gardens near the Felsenreitschule opera house that is literally built into the mountainside. Our photographer took some really neat pictures throughout the gardens. These are the same gardens that Julie Andrews and the children dance around in singing "Do-Re-Me" in the 1965 movie.

The photographer posed us for one particular picture. We faced one another on the cobblestone walkway of Old Town Salzburg. Our eyes locked and filled with tears. We were having such a wonderful trip, such a wonderful time celebrating Scott's birthday. The love we felt for each other at that moment was powerful. There it was, pure and simple love, right in front of me. If I hadn't known before that moment that this man truly loved me, I knew for sure then. It was like lightning had just struck. I sometimes had wondered, as the years passed, whether or not Scott really loved me. I had experienced so much heartbreak and disappointment in my life. I admit that over the twenty years we'd been together, I had moments when I took our relationship for granted. Not any more. The look in his eyes, that moment, told me everything I needed to know. His eyes were filled with so much love and devotion.

That look was just like the one he gives me today. It's a look that paralyzes you when you see it. It's pure and real. It's the look of true love.

My dearest Scott,

I want to thank you for your love, devotion and all that you do to help and support me every single day. I feel your love every minute. You are the love of my life. Thanks to you, I know what true love is. I want you to know here and now that if the day comes when I pass, I do not want you to ever think there was more you could have or should have done. You're doing it. You are the love of my life. Our life together has been a fairy tale of many dreams come true. I want you to know that I do notice all of what you do, especially the little things. For all the time we've had together, it's the time since my diagnosis that means the most to me. Every single day we've had together has meant the world to me. I love you.

—*Your Louis, always and forever . . .*

Thursday, November 14

Scott and I pause and step back as we talk about the future and discuss some decisions we need to make sooner rather than later. For as much as we've already been through, our relationship continues to be tested more and more. The fear of the unknown weighs heavy on us. We reinforce our commitment to get through this extreme challenge. My cancer is doing what cancer does: growing. I remind myself this is only another one of life's speed bumps. A temporary setback. This cancer has no idea who it is dealing with. Scott and I remain confident that we will continue to power through to meet this challenge. More importantly, we truly believe what we've always believed: we will overcome this cancer. Nothing can beat the power of love.

Friday, November 15

It's been a crazy week given the news from my CT scan. This day mirrors most of the other days this week. No real change with my pain. My overall energy level this week has been okay. Scott and I developed a per-day schedule last week for what household chores need to be done in order to get ready for our party on Saturday. We adopt the one-day-at-a-time slogan as we move forward.

I am not comfortable walking away from Keytruda as per Dr. CO's recommendation for today's ninth cycle. Fortunately, Dr. CO supported my decision to keep Keytruda in addition to Alimta for my treatment dose today. Scott and I begin to wonder, as we are literally driving to the cancer center to receive this treatment, if we should also add carboplatin back in, since it seems that the cancer returned after my first four treatment cycles when carboplatin was used. The Keytruda/Alimta plus carboplatin triplet is the one defined in the Keynote-189 study protocol. We hope Dr. CO will support our decision. With carboplatin being the powerhouse of the three drugs, Scott and I believe that adding carboplatin back into my treatment this cycle could slow down the cancer while we look to begin the EGFR-targeted agent: Tagrisso. This, along with the fact that I had great results when I was on the triplet of drugs during my first four Keytruda Combo treatment cycles, supports our thought process.

As we are driving and discussing my treatment, I receive a text from Kyle, my previous manager at Merck. He asks if carboplatin is being added back. We're in sync! I share with him that I already reached out to Dr. Langer last night to run this by him and get his thoughts. Unfortunately, I haven't heard back from Dr. Langer yet. Fortunately, Dr. CO supports our decision to add carboplatin back in. I will receive the Keytruda/Alimta and carboplatin today. Scott and I are happy with this decision.

While I am in the infusion chair getting ready to receive my IV treatment, my phone rings with a 215 area code. It's Dr. Langer! I tell him that I'm actually in the infusion chair and that I have asked Dr. CO to re-initiate the Keytruda Combo that includes all three drugs. Dr. Langer fully supports this decision, and we immediately discuss initiating the EGFR drug Tagrisso as soon as possible. Our plan is to start Tagrisso by the end of the first week of December after my medical appointments that week. The clock is ticking; there's no time to wait. Three weeks will have to be sufficient. After our meeting with Dr. CO, prior to receiving my treatment today, Scott and I discussed that it might be best to have Dr. Langer become my primary oncologist. Given Dr. Langer's breadth and depth of experience, along with my recent disease progression, Scott and I believe that this is the best decision for everyone. We will tell each doctor at my next appointment with them.

In the afternoon, I'm working from home and have a one-on-one with my manager. I received good feedback from my peers on my presentations this week. Many coworkers expressed their support and offered to do whatever is needed to support my workload. The term "hero" was used. This warms my heart.

After a long day and emotionally exhausting week, Scott and I are very excited today as Caro and Dano are flying in for our Celebration event. They will be staying with us and have offered to help out any way they can with the party. Scott and I have stayed on track with our chore schedule all week, but there are a few things left to be done. Having Caro and Dano here will be so helpful. They arrive about 7 PM, and we order Italian takeout and enjoy catching-up with our dear friends.

§

We first met Caro and Dano in the fall of 2015, just prior to when I started my new position at Merck. Scott and I were attending the yearly black-tie Rubicon vintage launch party at Francis and Eleanor Coppola's Inglenook winery in Napa Valley, California. Rubicon is Inglenook's flagship premium wine. It's a Napa Valley super red. It's Scott's and my favorite!

Scott and I had attended several Rubicon events in the past. We always had the time of our lives. This event would be no different. We were seated at a round-top table of eight, and Caro and Dano sat across from us. I immediately noticed Caro in her beautiful Amani-style navy blue gown. Her husband, Dano, wore an elegant black-tie tuxedo. The type you'd see James Bond wearing. Like Scott and I, Caro and Dano celebrate life to its fullest. There was an immediate connection between the four of us. Dano was referring to his wife as "Caro" that night. Scott and I thought that was cool, and I immediately took that a step further as a homage to *Hawaii Five-O* and called Dan "Dano." Since that night, Scott and I fondly refer to them as our dear friends, Caro and Dano.

During our dinner, Scott and I shared that we were getting legally married that November during a ceremony in our home. Dano was very interested and asked if they could attend. This struck me, given that we had just met them. I could tell by his interest, along with his enthusiasm for us, that he was genuine. After dinner, I excused myself to go to the restroom. I saw Caro on the way back. There was a five-piece jazz band, and Caro asked me what we're doing next. Without hesitation, I said we were going outside to visit with Francis Ford Coppola. He likes to sit outside after dinner and smoke cigars on the terrace, under the Italian lights. This would be a great opportunity to meet him. Caro looked puzzled and responded that she and Dano ran regularly and didn't smoke cigars. I said that's okay we don't smoke either, and we run regularly as well. But if you want to meet Francis Ford Coppola, this is the time to do so. Her eyes widened, and off we went to visit with Mr. Coppola. We had a great time and were even more thrilled when Eleanor came out. At first, I believe she came to get Francis and return home, as it was late. But after we gave her such a warm welcome, she stayed to visit with us past midnight. That wonderful evening launched an enduring friendship with Caro and Dano.

....

Saturday, November 16

Our Celebration of Life, Love and Friendship Event is today!!! Scott and I have been waiting for this day for months. Even more so despite the disappointing news. Caro, Dano, Scott and I all wake up early and begin last-minute preparations to get ready for our guests to arrive at 2 PM. The Ice Sculpture is the first to arrive at 12:45 PM. It's a re-creation of the LOVE sign in downtown Phila-delphia. The sculpture looks *awesome*, complete with LED light-ing that illuminates the ice. It is larger than we expected. Amidst the excitement of deliveries, the catering team and flowers arrive. The flowers are beautiful, jewel tone colors, similar to the flowers we selected for our 25th anniversary celebration, and well worth the audacious price tag. It is a bit frantic, but everything comes together.

Scott and I pause to sit together as Helen, our friend and harpist from Curtis, plays Bach's Prelude no. 1 from the Well-Tempered Clavier, BMV 846. I'd like to share with you one of my favorite recordings of this piece.[35] Listening to this music tells you everything there is to know about the love that is here today. This day belongs to all of our dear friends who have supported Scott and me from day one of my diagnosis. Not cancer. Dr. Langer graciously accepted our invitation to attend and speak about my journey. I am so happy to see him and meet his dear wife, Mindy. My friends and coworkers Mare, Carolyn and Kyle share some kind words. I am honored to have Dr. Langer give a compelling speech on my behalf. He mentions that he's not used to these types of events where the patient is present. He has a catchphrase: "By hook or by crook, we'll get Louis to the top of the Kaplan-Meier curve." To make our day more special, Carolyn made a huge banner that we hang up on the loft ledge overlooking the family room: *Celebrating Louis 2.0.*

The entire evening is surreal. I'm so happy to see everyone, but I am overwhelmed by the crowd. My back pain is so bad that I find myself avoiding our guests so as to prevent long periods of standing. I feel terrible doing this, but as I walk around, I'm thrilled to see all my friends and coworkers having a good time. By the end of the evening, I am exhausted but uplifted by all the love that was shared tonight. It is a memory Scott and I will cherish forever.

[35.] *Music:* Lang Lang piano performance of Bach: Prelude from the Prelude and Fugue in C Major, BWV 846 in The Well-Tempered Clavier: Book 1 (YouTube video, 2:20). Posted by Deutsche Grammophon, June 21, 2019; accessed September 2020. *https://www.youtube.com/watch?v=7ZNXBpO-uEo*

Sunday, November 17

I'm having a rough day. I definitely overdid it yesterday. My overall energy level is around 20 percent. Though I truly am emotionally, physically and mentally exhausted, I relish the thought that yesterday really did happen. I'm so glad Scott and I decided to do this, although it took all the energy I had to ensure everyone had a good time. The timing couldn't have been better. Once again, I am experiencing a nadir from having carboplatin back in my treatment. This was to be expected. Exhaustion aside, with all that is going on with my health, I am very happy that I was able to be with all our friends during our Celebration event yesterday. I'm so glad that Dano and Caro are still here. They truly have been a godsend. Scott and I couldn't have pulled off this weekend without them. We have bonded with them on a whole new level. Caro is our sister, and Dano is our brother.

This morning instead of showers, Scott and I take a bubble bath! Typically, we almost always take one together. This time I go first, so that I can stretch out and relax. I feel faint as I am getting out of the bathtub. Scott guides me over to our bed, where I lie down to catch my breath and relax. I am hyperventilating. I am scared. I start rambling. I tell Scott how much I love him and how I want him to go on and live a happy life. I tell him not to worry about me. I want him to go on his business trip to Raleigh, North Carolina. I tell him to knock his presentation out of the park! I will be okay. Dano will be here with me. Scott responds, saying not to worry and that I don't have to say all those things. I can see the worry in his loving eyes. It reminds me of that other look in his eyes, the one I saw in Salzburg, which makes me calm and happy.

Noon approaches and Caro is packing to leave for the airport. She needs to leave today for Charlotte. Scott shares with all of us as we sit on our family room sofa that he is canceling his business trip to Raleigh and wants Dano to leave with his wife, together.

Dano, Caro and I are shocked! Scott hasn't done this before. I am surprised, but very happy that Scott will be here with me.

With all that we've experienced together over the past twenty-six years, here we are facing our greatest fear of having less time together. Regardless of how scared I might be at times, I am so happy that I am the one with cancer, not Scott. I would be devastated if it were him. I would fall on the sword for him in a heartbeat. He is the love of my life. I love him with all my heart and soul.

....

Monday, November 18

I wake up feeling better. If I had to put a percentage on it, it would be about 60 percent. This is dramatically up from yesterday. I've been thinking about our friend Victoria ever since Scott shared with me how upset she was at our Celebration event. I wish I'd known this during the party. I would have comforted her, dried her tears and given her a great big hug to assure her that everything would be okay. I work most of the day today without a break. Victoria comes by to visit. I'm so glad to be able to give her that hug!

....

Tuesday, November 19

Today I speak with my Merck patient advocate and friend, Dr. Linda. The Keytruda U.S. Medical Team has invited me to share my journey. Dr. Linda is the point person for any internal request for me to share my cancer journey. She can tell by our conversation that I'm not feeling well and offers to cancel our portion of the event. At first I tell her that I am okay to continue with our plans. As the day goes on, however, I rethink my decision and decide that I shouldn't push it. Even though a driver was being arranged, the emotional drain from sharing my journey will exhaust me more. I reach out to Dr. Linda to let her know. She understands and is totally supportive. I am relieved as right now it's best to keep any additional stress at a minimum.

I hear from my good friend Margaret today! She stops by after work to visit. I always appreciate our time together. Margaret is a special friend. We met at work, three years ago. Margaret was at Scott's and my twenty-fifth anniversary celebration last year at Inglenook. It was a wonderful celebration. I most likely already had metastatic non-small cell lung cancer then. I'm so glad we didn't know. It would have ruined our celebration. I'm happy Margaret was there. Here's one of my favorite stories about her. At our twenty-fifth anniversary celebration, Scott and I gave all of our guests a 375-ml bottle of Rubicon as a party token. Margaret left our party and went directly to the San Francisco airport for an early morning flight. No sleep for her! On her way, she stopped at a 7-Eleven store and got a churro. Margaret opened the bottle of Rubicon wine using her car key. There she was, sitting near the San Francisco International airport, enjoying a churro with a 375-ml bottle of Rubicon in a bag. I love this story!

Tomorrow is Scott's and my twenty-sixth anniversary. Who knows what the future holds? If this ends up being our last anniversary together, I want to be together all day.

....

Wednesday, November 20

Happy anniversary to us! Scott and I met twenty-six years ago today on my mom's birthday. She would have been eighty-two years old today. I'm having a good day today. I am less fatigued with no nausea. My appetite has returned, and I'm able to eat several small meals throughout the day. We still have leftovers from our party, so there's plenty to eat.

§

As I mentioned, last year Scott and I threw a big anniversary party in Napa Valley! Twenty of our closest friends were invited to join us at the Inglenook winery. In 1975, Francis and Eleanor Coppola purchased the original 1879 Inglenook winery owned and built by Gustave Niebaum. The barrel room upstairs is where we celebrated. What a celebration for one of the happiest days of our life together. It took almost a year to plan. There was one large, long "king's" table. Scott and I sat in the middle with all our friends seated around us. The celebration theme was post-World War II Hawaii. We love that era and we love Hawaii. Other than Venice, Italy, Hawaii is our second favorite place to travel. We have a lot of special memories there. Scott and I were dressed in black formal wear with ivory vests and long ivory ties so that we could look our best for pictures. We wanted our guests to be more comfortable, so all the men wore suits or sport jackets with no tie and the women wore dresses. Some of the women wore circa-1950s dresses to go with our post-World War II theme! We love Hawaiian flowers, so there were plenty of flowers streaming from above, almost covering the full length of the table—orchids, anthurium, hibiscus, birds of paradise and ginger. Their fragrance was magnificent! Everyone gasped when we entered the room for the grand reveal. Each table setting had no less than five wine glasses, one for each tasting and vintage year of wine.

The band was Steve Lucky and the Rhumba bums, who also performed at a Rubicon launch dinner that we attended back in 2007. They have a 1950s band vibe. They are a totally awesome six-piece band complete with Steve on piano, two saxophones, a drummer, bass player and guitarist Carmen Getit, who rocked it on her vintage '59 Gibson Epiphone guitar.

Scott and I arranged to have a photographer take pictures. He was highly recommended by our winery event planner, Matthew. The photographer was expensive. I remember when we were negotiating, I believed the price we were getting was based on a wedding. I kept saying how small the event was, that there were no children and it wasn't a wedding. Not that this means anything. I was thinking that having no children at the party would carry some sort of savings. What do I know? Throughout the negotiation process, the photographer stayed firm. Then I remembered what friends had shared with us about photographers: you get what you pay for.[36] So, there it was. The pictures were put all together in a video format, complete with music. It told the story of our special evening from beginning to end. Francis Ford Coppola's personal assistant was with us and had arranged to have the entrance road closed until we finished our pictures. Scott and I remember the walkie-talkie call that was made, as we were en route to the front gate, instructing a crew to remove the vineyard equipment as it would have appeared in the background of our photos. At the entrance gate, our photographer positioned us for our first photo. Scott and I stood facing each other, just as we did in Salzburg. I saw that same look in his eyes. I had tears flowing down my cheeks as our eyes connected. Twenty-five years went by so fast. It seemed like just yesterday that we first met!

Scott's ninety-two-year-old Aunt Shirley was there along with his brother, Mark, and sister-in-law, Alison. His cousin Helena passed away from pancreatic cancer the year prior, but her husband, Marco, was able to join us along with his daughter, Merissa, Scott's great cousin, and Merissa's husband, Chris. Marco lives in Walnut Creek, California, in the same home that he and Helena lived in together. He is celebrating his birthday today! Merissa and Chris live in Seattle, Washington. They were able to attend with their new baby, Antonia. She is absolutely adorable! She looks just like the Gerber baby. Antonia was only six months old at the time, but nothing was going to stop them from joining our celebration. I've known Merissa since she started her theater major at UC Irvine back in the '90s. Scott and I are so happy that they are able to join us!

[36.] Our friends were right! If you're looking for a great photographer in the San Francisco Bay Area, please contact Alex and Anastasia Zyuzikov at *www.redspherestudios.com.*

Caro and Dano were there, of course, along with Scott's friend Shawn and his new wife, Grace. Scott's longtime friend and ex-coworker, Andreas, was able to make it all the way from London. He brought Samia. Scott and I thought she was his date, but they announced they'd recently been married. We were thrilled to hear the wonderful news! Samia was one of the women who wore a circa-1950s outfit. She defined the era perfectly! Candice and her brother Joe flew in from North Carolina and Ohio. They both looked great! Joe donned a fedora, which added a hint of the *Godfather* theme to the evening. Another one of Scott's ex-coworkers, Ben, and his wife, Lydia, from the Bay Area completed our invite list. It was a once in a lifetime celebration! Scott and I had the time of our lives![37]

Thursday, November 21

I was able to eat a lot yesterday, which was more than I've been able to eat lately due to nausea. Because of this, I went to the bathroom several times throughout the night. I wake up weak from diarrhea. I must be dehydrated. Sorry, I know this sounds gross, but this helps describe the ups and downs of dealing with cancer. I end up drinking a lot of water and take a long nap at lunchtime. Scott is so sweet. He goes to the store while I am napping to get some chicken noodle soup. I am so happy! I love chicken noodle soup! Although I am nauseous, this is one meal I'll never turn down. I am able to eat almost all of the large container. The soup is nice and hot, just bland enough to be delicious and fill me up.

I have fond memories of my mom staying home from work to be with me when I was sick. She'd go to the store and get some ginger ale and Donald Duck orange juice. I remember the smell

---

[37.] Scott and I would like to share our special 25th anniversary video with you. Here is the YouTube link. Enjoy! *https://www.youtube.com/watch?v=gs6lGgQSnHU&t=3s*

of her perfume, Chanel No. 5, as she felt my forehead to see if the fever was gone.

....

Friday, November 22

My energy is coming back. I'm at about 70 percent with no pain or discomfort. I slept well. I'm looking forward to enjoying a relaxing, uneventful weekend with Scott. The weather is cooler. Each day has been around 45°F. Autumn is definitely here. This week reminds me of my first week of Keytruda Combo back at the end of May. The big difference this time is that at least 60 percent of the overall cancer in my body is gone. I am hopeful that making the decision to add back in carboplatin to Keytruda and Alimta was the right decision. Scott and I have every confidence that by reinitiating Keytruda Combo we'll regain some ground, or at the very least, keep the cancer from growing any more.

....

Saturday, November 23

My energy continues to return. I feel about 85 percent with no pain and little nausea. Scott and I have a good day together. We discuss our Orient Express trip in April to celebrate my sixtieth birthday! Contingent on my ability to travel during that time, we decide our alternative option will be to stay locally in downtown Philadelphia at the new Four Seasons Hotel in the newly built Comcast Tower, the highest building in downtown Philly. We always enjoy our time in downtown Philadelphia. It's a big city, but not so big that it's hard to get around. The new "W" hotel also opens in January. We discuss this option as well. We have great alternatives to our initial trip plans for Venice, Paris and the Orient Express.

I'm able to join Scott to run some errands today. It is nice to get outside! I enjoy walking up and down the aisles in the grocery store. At check-out I decide to take it easy, so I ask Scott for the car keys to go back to the car to relax.

Sunday, November 24

I continue to feel better with more energy. I'm somewhere around 85 percent energy level.

It's been a while since we connected with our good friend Candice. She had a birthday earlier this month. Scott and I have been waiting for the right time to tell Candice and her brother Joe about my lung cancer. We met Candice back in 2014, in Dayton, Ohio, at a wine tasting inside our local Kroger grocery store. Candice was sitting near us enjoying her wine when she overheard Scott and me talking about Far Niente wines. She mentioned how much she loved Far Niente, and we've been good friends ever since.

Soon after meeting Candice, she invited us over to her home. During that visit, we met Joe for the first time. He was quiet at first, but warmed up to Scott and me as the night went on. Joe is a great guy. He has a great sense of humor and a big heart to go with it. We consider Candice and Joe family. They've been close friends ever since we met, which makes it more difficult to tell them about my cancer.

Candice lived about half a mile from where we lived, in a historic Waynesville home built circa 1844. Yes, it's haunted. It's a cool home. It's got a nice vibe. Not all ghosts are bad. You literally feel something present in certain areas as you walk through the house, especially in the upstairs front bedroom! In the basement, you can see where tunnels were dug to support the Underground Railroad during the Civil War.

Candice's partner of many years passed away from melanoma cancer a few years ago. Scott and I can tell by the way she spoke about AJ that she loved him very much. Candice is a doctor. In early 2016 she moved to North Carolina to take a physician position at a community practice so that she could be closer to her sister and brother-in-law in a community near the beach. Our call today goes well. It is great seeing Candice via FaceTime. We don't want to make our call a downer, so Scott and I decide to wait to share the news about my cancer.

....

Monday, November 25

I've been sneezing a lot over the past few days. Scott and I are concerned that I'm coming down with a cold. Last night, my sneezing increased. It's definitely a cold. I'm lightheaded with less energy today. Perhaps my cold is causing me to feel lightheaded. I'm feeling chilled so I put on a long-sleeved shirt, long johns and two pairs of socks. My feet have been feeling cold. This is probably a side effect of the carboplatin. Carboplatin belongs to a group of drugs called "platinums." Cold hands and feet can be a side effect of platinum drugs. Despite my cold, I am comfortable with little pain and mild nausea. I am happy that I feel well enough to write about my day!

....

Tuesday, November 26

Thanksgiving is Thursday! I'm at about 70 percent energy level. I'm feeling better today, though I continue to feel lightheaded. I have a little pain with some fatigue, which accounts for my lack of energy. I have an appointment in advance of my follow-up MRI of the brain and spine scheduled for tomorrow at the Abington-Jefferson Blair Mill Road Radiology Center. I haven't had a brain or spine MRI since August, so today we get to see where I'm at.

Our dear friend Alisha stops by after Scott and I return home from the Radiology Center. We always enjoy seeing Alisha. We debrief on our Celebration event. Our hour-long visit passes quickly. Time always goes by fast when we see Alisha. She is very positive and always has a beautiful smile that is certain to make everyone feel better. I am reminded how much I love her laugh and sense of humor.

I practice my horn today. It's been challenging lately with my pain, nausea and fatigue, but I've kept to my daily practice schedule as best I can. I rarely miss a day. It really motivates me.

....

Wednesday, November 27

Thank goodness for Mozart! The Clarinet Concerto in A Major, K 662 and the Flute and Harp Concerto in C Major, K 299 are a couple of the Mozart pieces playing in my headset during my brain and spine MRIs. I am in that machine for almost two hours. Initially, I was in another MRI machine, apparently a newer model. After several attempts by the technician, the machine would not start. About fifteen minutes in, and yes, I was in the machine while George was trying to start it, we switched to another machine. Apparently, this is an older model because when we go from the spine imaging to the brain, I have to get up while the panels and headset are changed. Although I appreciate the break from being inside the "tube," it is very annoying. I'm claustrophobic, so that doesn't help. I just want this to be over with.

George shares that he is going to increase the time for my brain scan by an additional five minutes in order to get more detailed imaging since I have a prior history of brain tumors, from back when I was first diagnosed with three small brain metastases. We arrived at the Blair Mill Road radiology imaging center at 8:30 AM. My appointment was for 9:15 AM. Fortunately, since it was early and the Wednesday before Thanksgiving, I was called to the back right at 9:15 AM. By the time we switch machines and complete my MRI, it is noon.

Scott is wonderful! Once George lets him know my appointment is running overtime, he goes to Wawa to get breakfast sandwiches and coffee for us.

Poor Scott had pink/red color around both eyes when he woke up this morning. It is the first thing I notice when I come out to the lobby after my MRIs. I am also experiencing some "sand" coming out of my right eye. Scott definitely has pink eye. His is full-blown and mine is just starting. We are a mess! Never before have we had health issues. We both are scared about my cancer, and this added eye issue doesn't help.

Exhausted, I take a nap as soon as we get home. At 2 PM, I receive a phone call from Dr. CO. Once again, I can always tell by the tone of their voice when it isn't good news. Receiving a call from your oncologist the same day as a CT scan is never good news in my experience. I feel myself freeze in place and brace: my brain MRI identified thirteen metastases in my brain. Most are very small, but one is 1.5 cm. Needless to say, I am stunned. It is immediately apparent that my EGFR Exon 19 mutation caused my cancer to start growing again. Apparently, as soon as I finished the four treatment cycles of Keytruda Combo and dropped the carboplatin, my cancer reversed course and began to grow.

There is mild swelling around the 1.5-cm lesion located in the middle of the left lobe of my brain. It is not near any vital areas and is considered "small." Dr. CO recommends I start a steroid to reduce the swelling. I will begin taking the same dexamethasone that I take around my cycles, only now I'll take it daily until the swelling stops. I have a thirty-day supply on hand, and Dr. CO recommends that I take 2 mg in the morning and 2 mg at the end of the day, at 4 PM, for a total of 4 mg per day. This shouldn't keep me up at night. Dexamethasone will help reduce the swelling in my brain. I need to be on the lookout for symptoms caused by the swelling: loss of feeling on one side and corollary inability to walk, falling, and headaches. Fortunately, I'm not experiencing any of these symptoms.

Scott comes over as soon as he hears that I am on the phone with Dr. CO. I share the news with Scott while I'm on the call. We both are visibly shaken. If the swelling continues and I become symptomatic, I will need to go to the ER right away. They would perform a full brain radiology treatment to reduce the swelling. This radiation could affect my cognitive function, which would be reflected in some memory loss. Scott and I look at each other as I talk on the phone. We're both scared to death.

Dr. CO remains optimistic and has already started the prior authorization process with our health insurance company to obtain my Tagrisso. Because of the cost of this medication, it needs to be administered by a specialty pharmacy. The specialty pharmacy will monitor refills and deliver the medication monthly via FedEx. I ask Dr. CO to share my MRI results with Dr. Langer prior to December 3 so we can discuss this information at my next appointment.

Tagrisso, produced by AstraZeneca, is a third-generation TKI. It is a once-a-day pill that I will take every day, most likely for the rest of my life. Tagrisso crosses the blood-brain barrier into the brain.[38] That is a good thing in this case. Its pharmacokinetic activity has an affinity to shrink or destroy brain metastasis.[39] My brain metastases need to be treated now before they get bigger.

Side effects may include decreased appetite, rash, QTc interval changes (heart stuff), lightheadedness and the feeling that you might pass out, and decreased lung function. I will need to power through these side effects as this pill will determine the duration of the rest of my life. Dr. CO believes that three weeks is sufficient time to allow for a washout period between my last Keytruda dose and the beginning of starting Tagrisso. As previously mentioned, this washout period is very important as any Keytruda remaining

---

[38.] The blood-brain barrier serves as a filter, controlling which molecules can pass from the blood into the brain. Because the endothelial cells are positioned so closely together, they keep out any harmful toxins or pathogens from reaching your brain. *Source: https://www.verywellhealth.com/search?q=blood+brain+barrier*

[39.] Please refer to the FDA-approved package insert for Tagrisso at *www.tagrisso .com/* for details on Tagrisso's activity on patients with brain metastasis. The Flaura study provided the clinical information that supported the new-drug FDA indication for Tagrisso for first-line treatment of metastatic non–small cell lung cancer patients who are EGFR positive.

in my body poses the risk of causing side effects with the EGFR medication. If Dr. Langer agrees with this timeline, I will be starting Tagrisso as soon as possible after my December 3 appointment with him. In the meantime, I will be relaxing and doing all I can to think positive.

I hang up the phone. I do not cry. There's no time for that. I immediately jump back into survival mode and focus on what we can do to eliminate these tumors in my brain. Scott and I talk about it and are very confident that Tagrisso will work. I feel comfort soon after starting dexamethasone. Once again, Scott and I discuss that it's time to make Dr. Langer my primary oncologist. In the past, Dr. CO communicated "bad news" as if it meant the end was near. I believe this is through no fault of their own; Dr. CO is a new oncologist. There are more options today for treating stage 4 non-small cell lung cancer that can prolong survival than there were twenty years ago. With these options, a new oncologist sometimes has less experience communicating bad news. An experienced oncologist is able to communicate more optimistically based on having less treatments available throughout their career. Disease progression makes my treatment moving forward that much more important. All of this is why Scott and I made our decision.

Thursday, November 28

Happy Thanksgiving! Scott and I have a lot to be thankful for regardless of the news yesterday. After all, I AM STILL HERE!!! Cancer can kiss my ass! I'm not going anywhere, anytime soon. I woke up feeling great, and I'm close to 100 percent energy level, which is the best I've felt in weeks. It truly is a great day! Scott went to the store and got all the fixings to support a traditional Thanksgiving dinner. He selected a "young" turkey that only includes the breast, which, we agree, is the best part! Maple syrup and vanilla-flavored yams are delicious! The turkey is nice and tender—perfect! Candied cranberries, gravy and homemade stuffing complete the meal. It is a wonderful dinner!

During dinner we listen to Mozart Piano Concertos nos. 20, 22, 24 and 25. The house is lit up and filled with the smell of fresh turkey baking. I have a good practice on my horn, which makes me very happy. *Jurassic Park* was on TV earlier this morning. Scott and I love the horn music from that soundtrack. I couldn't wait to play those same themes on my horn during my practice session tonight. Today is exactly what we needed after all the news yesterday. It is a wonderful day, a very special Thanksgiving!

Friday, November 29

I wake up at 4:45 AM, wide awake. I play *Solitaire* on my iPhone. This helps make me sleepy enough to go back to bed an hour later. I am able to sleep until 7:30 AM. Fatigue is back, and my energy level returns to about 70 percent. It's okay though, because I am able to do some writing. I am determined to get better. I beat cancer with my initial treatment, and I have every intention of doing the same now. The EGFR-targeted therapy Tagrisso should be exactly what I need to target my Exon 19 mutation and kill the cancer. I look forward to starting this treatment soon.

At 2 PM, I receive a call from the on-call community oncologist covering for Dr. CO today. Scott and I are alerted. By now, we know that it isn't good news when the doctor calls, especially the day after Thanksgiving. Once again, I brace myself. The on-call oncologist shares the results from the MRI on my spine, in particular the T10 area of my spine where the cancer had been before. The lesion near my spine fracture at T10 has grown. The doctor asks if I've experienced urinary/intestinal incontinence or numbness in my feet. I respond that at least one day during the week I have a tingling, pinched-nerve feeling down my left leg that is bothersome and annoying. They say that this is related to the pressure the lesion is causing on my spine and ask if I've felt dizzy or lightheaded. I say yes, that I purposefully have to get my bearings whenever I go to stand and begin walking. The doctor says this is also attributed to the pressure on my spine. We agree to increase the steroid dose from 4 to 6 mg per day to address the tingling in my feet.

The on-call oncologist recommends that I go to the ER because, based on the size of the tumor on my spine and the pressure it's causing, I may have urinary incontinence and/or numbness in my legs that will affect my ability to walk. I say I am fine. My ability to urinate is normal and I can walk. I'm not going to the ER. I think to myself that nothing will happen there given that it's Thanksgiving weekend. I will be more comfortable here at home with Scott given the fact that I have no symptoms. The ER is for people who need the ER. I assure the oncologist that I will go to the ER if any of these symptoms occur. The doctor recommends that I initiate a visit with a radiologist next week to schedule radiation treatment to my spine in the T10 area. I agree to do this. I would receive radiation for ten days based on the radiologist's assessment and recommendation. We confirm that I should be able to have my EGFR drug Tagrisso next week. As I mentioned, Tagrisso will immediately begin to address my brain lesions and the radiation will address my back pain and peripheral neuropathy, meaning the tingling in my feet. I am inspired, despite the bad news, as I feel empowered being in the solution. This is all good information because it provides important treatment solutions in crucial areas.

Saturday, November 30

I wake up at 2:45 AM, wide awake, due to the dexamethasone. The increased dexamethasone dose definitely will be keeping me up at night. After getting back to sleep, I wake up a few hours later feeling better. The shooting pain down my left leg is gone. Now I feel pain through both sides of my buttocks, which makes sitting down uncomfortable. To avoid this, I shift from lying down on one side to the other. Scott and I enjoy a quiet day together watching movies on Netflix. I drift in and out of sleep with short catnaps during the movies.

Scott and I are excited that our friends Melissa and JC are coming by tonight. They offered to pick up takeout from one of our favorite restaurants, Basta Pasta in Skippack. They arrive right on time at 6 PM. We spend the next couple hours catching up and revisiting the moments of our Celebration event. Teary-eyed, I fill them in on the news of my latest MRIs and the plan for treatment going forward. Melissa and I worked together supporting Keytruda, so she is familiar with Tagrisso's use for EGFR-positive lung cancer patients. I share with Melissa and JC that based on my disease progression, I will begin the EGFR Tagrisso by the end of the first week in December, once I've seen Dr. Langer that week.

During our visit, Melissa and JC agree with our decision to move Dr. Langer to be my primary oncologist. Scott and I share that we will tell Dr. CO at my next appointment. Making this move was always an option. With all that's occurred lately, this seems to be the best way to support my treatment path moving forward. Melissa and JC recall Dr. Langer speaking at our Celebration event. They heard what I shared and what Dr. Langer shared on my behalf. They absolutely believe that with all my knowledge on oncology, specifically lung cancer, coupled with Dr. Langer's expertise, that together we will make shared, well-thought-out decisions for my treatment. Hearing Melissa and JC saying it out loud is just what we needed.

Melissa and I share a special connection. We've always believed there is a type of clairvoyance between us. Melissa's and JC's son Jack was born on my birthday, April 22. During our visit today, Melissa shares that JC grew up on a street named "Stockton," and that the word Stockton has other significance in his life. To the extent that if they ever have another child who is a boy, his middle name will be Stockton. Scott and I also have a connection to a street named Stockton. How coincidental is that!

DECEMBER

....

Sunday, December 1

True to form, dexamethasone yet again keeps me awake at night. I wake up at 3:45 AM and am awake for an hour. I play *Solitaire* on my cell phone until I get tired. I go back to bed and sleep until 7:30 AM. I am glad, despite the sleep interruption, that I was able to fall back asleep and continue sleeping through the night. Today is the best I've felt since my last Keytruda Combo treatment in mid-November. My energy level is around 85 percent, and I have no pain, discomfort or nausea, with very little fatigue. Thank goodness I'm having a good day with all that's going on. I spend the day writing and preparing for my Tuesday appointment with Dr. Langer. During my Abington-Jefferson MRIs of the brain and spine, I asked for a CD so that Dr. Langer will be able to view my images at my next appointment, just in case he doesn't receive them. I believe that part of why I feel so good today is not solely because of the higher dose of dexamethasone I'm taking, but from the anti-cancer activity of adding back the carboplatin with Keytruda and Alimta.

Today I will be practicing my French horn before Scott and I leave for the Marriott Courtyard in Navy Yard in downtown Philadelphia. Scott has a business workshop tomorrow, and we will be staying overnight through Tuesday morning, when we go directly to my appointment with Dr. Langer across town at Penn Medicine. It will be nice to get away for a couple of days. No laundry or household chores, including making the bed and cleaning the shower. I'm taking my French Horn with me so I can practice while Scott is in meetings. I'll be working remotely while we're away.

Monday, December 2

I slept through the night last night—yeah! We checked in at the Marriott Courtyard yesterday at 3 PM. It's a nice hotel. Our room is spacious and clean, but there is no room service. We order Chinese food from one of our favorite restaurants in Philadelphia: Buddakan. Fortunately, they're able to provide delivery through Grubhub. The food arrives piping hot, nice and fresh. We enjoy their lobster fried rice. It is so delicious! Our bellies are full as we watch the end of *Jurassic Park* and all of *Jurassic Park 2* and then go to bed at 11 PM. We usually go to bed no later than 10:30 PM. I'm hoping that going to bed a little later will help me sleep through the night.

This morning I receive a voicemail at 8:27 AM from Dawn, the radiology scheduler with Abington-Jefferson, requesting that I come today at 10:30 AM today for an appointment with the radiologist. I call back immediately and am able to connect directly with Dawn. I share that it will not be possible, with such short notice, for me to get there today or tomorrow (I have my appointment with Dr. Langer tomorrow). Dawn turns over the call to Riley, the radiologist nurse practitioner. I repeat what I told Dawn regarding my availability. I let Riley know that Wednesday or Thursday, December 4 or 5, will work best. I also say that I'm fine and I don't believe this needs to be a fire drill. Riley says she is following up on a request from Dr. CO for me to see the radiologist ASAP, based on the report of the results from my spine MRI. They received the request the day after Thanksgiving. That's the same day I received a call from the on-call community oncologist. Riley says she will get right back to me.

Riley calls back at 9 AM and confirms a 1:30 PM appointment for Thursday, December 5. I laugh and mention that this truly isn't a fire drill, otherwise they would have gotten me in first thing in the morning on Wednesday, rather than Thursday. She is quick to mention that I was asked to go to the ER last Friday, based on the compression in my spine. I remind Riley that I was asymptomatic and preferred not to spend my Thanksgiving weekend in the hospital, and ask if she would have done the same under the same circumstances. She doesn't have a response. I ask for her to pass on a request to Dr. CO to have the MRI spine report from the radiologist uploaded to my patient portal for Abington-Jefferson so that I can see the results. Riley says that she typically doesn't have anything to do with the portal but will convey my message to Dr. CO. She accuses me of yelling at her. I am quick to let her know I wasn't yelling; I was actually smiling as I was listening to her remind me that I should have gone to the ER. I am confident in my response that this was not a fire drill. I often feel like a cow in line for a cattle call with how I'm treated by some medical personnel with all of their "go here," "go there" orders. It seems patronizing at times. This serves as a reminder for patients to set limits and not be simply at the mercy of the medical protocols.

....

Tuesday, December 3

I have my appointment with Dr. Langer today! I will be asking him to be my primary oncologist moving forward. I want to confirm this with him first before telling Dr. CO. After his gracious speech at our Celebration event, I believe that now is the best time to make this change as I transition from systemic chemotherapy and immunotherapy as my primary treatment to the EGFR Tagrisso so that we can address my Exon 19 mutation.

Dr. Langer does not hesitate to say yes when I ask him to be my primary oncologist. He immediately shares his plan, and together we review the results of my brain and spine MRI images. He reviews the symptoms that could occur as a result of the cancer returning. Cognitively, my motor skills could be affected, I could have decreased left/right coordination and numbness on either side. For my spine, my ability to walk could be affected, and I might experience incontinence. Happily, I still don't have any of these symptoms. I am completely asymptomatic.

At one point as Dr. Langer is explaining the possible side effects from the mild pressure caused by the 1.5-cm lesion in my brain, I look at him and say, "Dr. Langer, I play my French horn every day." He smiles and stops explaining symptoms, realizing that I am fine!

Quite honestly though, my spine MRI does not look good. Dr. Langer says I need radiation and if that were his spine, he'd be in traction! Based on the image, I should be having symptoms, but I do not. I attribute this to the many years of exercise and taking care of myself. Taking care of my body has given me the ideal foundation to withstand all that this cancer is throwing at me.

Dr. Langer and I discuss what our Plan C options are if Tagrisso and/or the radiation don't work. He mentions adding an angiogenesis inhibitor, Avastin, in addition to a platinum/taxane (Taxotere) combination. He says in that case I would lose my hair. I don't think so! I will stick with Alimta. Taxotere (docetaxel) is a cancer medicine that interferes with the growth and spread of cancer cells in the body. It is used to treat cancer of the breast, lung, prostate, stomach, and head/neck. Even though I sold Taxotere as an oncology sales representative, I prefer Alimta. I've already been on Alimta, and you don't lose your hair with Alimta. Since other options with carboplatin exist, I would prefer Alimta/carboplatin with Avastin versus generic Taxol or Taxotere. We'll see. I'm very hopeful that Tagrisso will be all we need.

On the way home, just as we are leaving Philadelphia, I receive a phone call from the specialty pharmacy. Tagrisso is a biologic and considered a high-value pharmacy drug. Specialty pharmacies typical manage distributing these types of drugs. They confirm that my Tagrisso will be sent out first thing tomorrow morning for delivery by noon, Thursday. So far, Scott and I have been very fortunate in regard to prescriptions costs, but with the monthly high cost of this drug we brace ourselves.

The pharmacy specialist confirms that the copay will be *zero*. I fight to hold the tears back. This is my life. This pill will determine my future no matter the cost. Later we receive documentation showing that this copay of zero is approved for one year. We are extremely grateful.

....

Wednesday, December 4

Scott and I enjoy a relaxing day as we reflect back on all that has taken place over the past month. We are happy that I will start Tagrisso tomorrow. This reinforces our belief that it all will work out. I am back on track, in the solution. My horn practice continues to serve as part of my physical therapy and is a wonderful distraction. I enjoy a good practice session today.

....

Thursday, December 5

I have my radiation preparation appointment at the Asplundh Cancer Center today at 1:30 PM. The goal of the radiation approach is to eliminate the lesion on my spine. "Dr. R," as I'll call him, will review my radiation treatment schedule to address the lesion that is causing mild pressure on my spine near the hairline fracture. Dr. Langer is very optimistic that this treatment will work and relieve the pressure and correct my spine.

Dr. R. is a very pleasant guy! Very positive and engaging. He says he likes my name, though "Louis Vincent Cesarini" prompted him to envision an older, taller man. He is surprised at how young I look. ☺ Needless to say, we get along very well! Dr. R says that I will receive ten sessions of radiation, each one lasting about ten minutes. Each treatment will focus on the exact area of the lesion. My spine will repair itself over the next few months. We look to schedule a spine MRI for mid-February to measure the progress.

Tagrisso is delivered at the end of the day. I take my first dose. As mentioned, the Flaura study is the registration study that gave Tagrisso its first-line FDA indication for EGFR-positive patients. The majority of patients in the Flaura study had the same Exon

19 mutation I have. All patients in the study were chemo-naïve, meaning they hadn't previously undergone chemotherapy. I, of course, am not. I was able to achieve about an 80 percent reduction in disease with Keytruda Combo. I am at about 70 percent reduction now. Tagrisso confronts less tumor burden today than it would have had otherwise if it had been used first. I believe that this fact can only increase the likelihood of a complete response. Additionally, the thirteen "small" brain metastases are more likely to go away faster, based on the blood-brain barrier affinity Tagrisso has. Our goal is to have the one 1.5-cm brain lesion that is causing "mild" pressure to go away or shrink by the time I have my next brain scan the first week of January. Our fingers are crossed.

Friday, December 6

We have my tenth infusion appointment with Dr. CO today. No infusion today! Although I've already started Tagrisso, we wanted to keep this appointment to review the image results from my brain and spine MRIs that I had the day before Thanksgiving.

As I share with Dr. CO that our preference is to have Dr. Langer become my primary oncologist, Scott and I can almost see the relief in Dr. CO's face. Certainly, this tells us that this is the best decision for everyone. Dr. CO shares with us that they were thinking about this last night. Scott and I are surprised to hear this. I sincerely thank Dr. CO for all the support and further that I hope our experience will help other lung cancer patients in some way. We part after a big hug accompanied by some tears.

So far, I'm not experiencing any side effects from Tagrisso.

Saturday, December 7

I feel good. Almost as if something is reconciling inside my body in a very good way. I'll take this as a good sign of what's to come!

Sunday, December 8

I continue to feel good. Some diarrhea but nothing else compelling. I have no pain, no fatigue and no nausea. My energy level is improving.

Monday, December 9

Radiation Day 1. My radiation treatment begins today. My friend Victoria graciously offered to drive me to and from my radiation appointments all this week, into next week. Before leaving, we enjoy a nice visit over coffee. Scott has an all-day workshop at an account at the Navy pier in downtown Philadelphia. He'll be able to take me to my appointments starting the end of next week.

As said, I'd been taking 2 mg of dexamethasone BID, meaning twice daily, which later increased to 4 mg BID with the news that the lesion on my spine had returned. I can tell you that this is a lot of steroid to take in one day. Each day, I feel my heart practically jumping out of my chest. It's the kind of feeling you get from being hyper-caffeinated or on a decongestant. Victoria laughs as I share my experience with dex and the fact that I probably shouldn't be drinking coffee! Tonight, as I have since late-November when I started steroids, I'm wide awake in the middle of the night. Once again, I play digital *Solitaire* on my iPhone until I feel tired enough to go back to sleep.

Tuesday, December 10

Radiation Day 2. We head to the cancer center for my second day of radiation treatment. So far, so good. I continue to practice my French horn daily, curious as to what effect, if any, this treatment has on my playing. This week, I can tell something is course-correcting in my spine. My ability to control my breathing while playing my horn is somewhat challenging. Since my lung cancer diagnosis, I classify my practice sessions as "high-school level," "early college," "senior-college level," and "professional." This week has more high-school level practice days based on my radiation treatment and the high dose of dexamethasone I am on. I remain patient, knowing that better practice sessions will come.

....

Wednesday, December 11

Radiation Day 3. Victoria and I allow extra time in the morning due to the snowy/rainy weather to get to my appointment. We discuss going to our Global team's holiday lunch celebration in Whitehouse Station, New Jersey, this coming Friday. We have asked Peter, Victoria's current manager and my previous manager, to drive us. I've rarely had this kind of quality time with Peter. Going with Peter to this holiday celebration has been something I've enjoyed and always looked forward to since I started at Merck. It's quality time that we otherwise might not have. We confirm with Peter that the three of us will be going together on Friday directly after my radiation treatment—yeah!

I have a check-in appointment with Dr. R directly following this third radiation treatment. He is happy to hear that I am not experiencing any nausea, weight loss or any discomfort and/or pain from the treatment so far. We discuss reducing my dexamethasone back down to 2 mg BID given the hyper feeling I've been experiencing. Dr. R agrees based on the lack of radiation-related side effects but says to wait until Monday to start reducing the dose. Needless to say, I'm happy to be able to lower my dex dose and reduce the hyper feeling. Perhaps I'll sleep better.

....

Thursday, December 12

Radiation Day 4. I make the decision to begin reducing my dexamethasone today instead of Monday. I can no longer stand the feeling of being so hyper! I want to have a good weekend and avoid waking up in the middle of the night. Meanwhile, I continue to feel great during my second week of Tagrisso. No nausea, no discomfort. The diarrhea is gone, and I'm more regular. I continue to take Senokot-S in the morning.

....

Friday, December 13

Radiation Day 5. I feel better already having reduced my dexamethasone down to 2 mg BID. I am sleeping better, thank goodness.

Victoria and I drive to Peter's home directly from my appointment. We all get into Peter's SUV and enjoy visiting and catching up with each other. The holiday party is great! I see many of my good friends and members of our leadership team. The venue is perfect! There are burning logs crackling in a large fireplace. White lights adorn the room to make the ambiance feel very festive. I sit with one of my BFFs, Erica, who drove up right next to us just as Peter was parking. It is great seeing Erica; she's so positive and extremely supportive. At our lunch table of ten, there is a pre-lit LED Christmas tree decorating our table. We learn that one person at each table has a raffle ticket underneath their coffee cup. This person will win the tree. That person is me! Everyone claps! It is the perfect way to top off our holiday celebration!

Scott had a workshop conference call that he was able to take from home. Additionally, a local designer was coming by to finish their install of our draperies in the living room, dining room, kitchen slider and master bedroom. We've been looking forward to this day since we started this project in June. Scott sent me pictures as it was completed. Everything looks stunning. The finished product is worth the wait.

....

Saturday-Sunday, December 14-15

Scott and I have a good weekend. I continue to feel better, ever since I cut my dexamethasone dose in half. I feel much less hyper. This is directly reflected in my horn playing, which begins to dramatically improve. I'm able to control my breathing much better than the previous week. Scott and I are in full holiday relaxation mode now. It's great to have time off to relax, spend time with Scott, and focus on getting better. Scott has totally unplugged and is no longer glued to his computer. I like when he does this. He works so hard.

Monday, December 16

Radiation Day 6. Victoria and I arrive at the cancer center in plenty of time. Scott is at all-day workshops in Collegeville. Good news! He finishes on Wednesday so he'll be able to take me to my radiation appointments on Thursday and Friday.

I really appreciate my time with Victoria this week. She is very supportive. We share stories of our lives that only reinforce the reason for our friendship.

Tuesday, December 17

Radiation Day 7. Victoria arrives early. She is so good about that. I continue to feel better. What a difference it makes being on a lower dexamethasone dose. My horn practicing continues to reflect this. Still no side effects from the Tagrisso. No pain, no fatigue, no nausea, no GI problems, sleeping well, eating great with 100 percent energy! Scott and I are so happy.

Wednesday, December 18

Radiation Day 8. I have my second check-in appointment with Dr. R directly following this eighth radiation treatment. I am excited to share with Dr. R that I have been feeling great and definitely can see improvement since my appointment with him a week ago. I share how the progress of my horn playing reflects this and that I am planning on recording the Beethoven Sonata in F Major, op. 17 for Horn and Piano soon. He asks for the YouTube link when it's posted.

Thursday, December 19

Radiation Day 9. Scott takes me to my radiation appointment today! They've been scheduled every day at 8:45 AM. We arrive early, as I always did with Victoria. I get my usual breakfast sandwich. Tuesdays and Thursdays, they have sausage-and-egg breakfast sandwiches, with egg and bacon on the other days. I always look forward to enjoying a cup of coffee and a breakfast sandwich while I visit with Victoria or Scott prior to my radiation appointment. What a great way to start the day!

Friday, December 20

Radiation Day 10. THIS IS THE FINAL DAY OF RADIATION!!! I'm glad that Scott is with me on my last appointment. All goes well. Patients get to ring a bell to announce the end of their radiation treatment. I do this with vigor! A radiation technician hands me a note from a young child in a school that supports cancer patients.

> *Hi, I am Tori, I'm from PA. I hope this make you happy. We are fighting with you. Everyone is fighting with you. You got this. We are cheering with you. Stay strong. Get well soon. People love you. I really hope you're a fighter.*
>
> *Love,*
> *Tori*

Well, Tori, if you read this, please know that I am a fighter and your note is so inspiring. I am doing very well as I continue my fight with lung cancer. I wish you, your family and friends good health and much happiness. No matter what life throws at you, know that you control your destiny and your attitude makes a world of difference. Thank you for all your love and support!

Your friend,
Louis

Saturday, December 21

We're off to see *The Nutcracker!* Scott and I made plans to attend this year's Pennsylvania Ballet annual production. We really didn't know if I would be well enough to make it at the time we bought our tickets. Certainly, we did not expect such a dramatic turnaround for the better having been on Tagrisso for three weeks now. Needless to say, we are thrilled that my health has taken such a 180-degree turn from where it was in mid-November at our Celebration of Life, Love and Friendship event. Scott and I are staying overnight at the Ritz Carlton. In true Ritz fashion, it's beautiful. It used to be an old bank building. The lobby has a full restaurant and bar. It has a great vibe. Our dear friend Lisa joins us. Lisa studied ballet when she was younger, into her high school years and beyond. Like us, she is a big *Nutcracker* enthusiast! What a wonderful experience for us to share.

The Pennsylvania Ballet George Balanchine production is fantastic![40] It includes a new Christmas tree, which they announce prior to the beginning of the performance. During the performance, the audience gasps when the tree begins to grow. The tree lights become more brilliant and begin to sparkle as the tree gets bigger! It is truly magnificent!

[40.] Tchaikovsky—The Nutcracker / De Notenkraker Yannick Nezet-Séguin and the Rotterdams Philharmonisch Orkest (YouTube video, 2:07:01). Please go to minute 29:24 when the Christmas tree begins to grow and minute 35:10 for when Clare and her Prince walk through the enchanted forest. Posted by NPO Radio 4, January 3, 2011, access by Louis Cesarini February 4, 2021. *https://www.youtube.com/watch?v=tk5Uturacx8*

Tchaikovsky—Western Ballet's The Nutcracker 2019 (YouTube video, 1:36:29). This program was aired on KMVT15 Community Media. Please go to minute 30:33 when the Christmas Tree begins to grow and minute 35:14 when the Prince and Clara meet and are escorted through the enchanted forest. Posted by KMVT December 13, 2019. Accessed February 4, 2021 by Louis Cesarini. *https://www.youtube.com/watch?v=lYayxixdeUs*

As I always do and certainly with more reason today, I make an unsuccessful attempt to keep the tears from rolling down my cheeks as the music swells and the tree rises. It is magical and overwhelming. The tears continue as the Snowflakes dance near the end of the first act. The music of Tchaikovsky here is quite powerful. Scott and I have premium box seats with plenty of room, in the first-level balcony with a perfect overhead view of everything on stage. It is truly spectacular! Lisa has a great seat as well in the upper orchestra section. We meet her at intermission and sip on a glass of champagne as we relive the highlights of Act I. The international dances of the second act are superb. There is an audible "ahh" as Marie and her prince fly away in a sled above the stage. What a great way to end the ballet! This is the best *Nutcracker* we've ever seen, a memory we will always cherish.

Afterward, Lisa joins us for a cocktail at the Ritz Carlton, and then we all enjoy a nice evening walk to Morimoto for dinner. Dinner is awesome; their sushi is the best! We have a wonderful time with Lisa, debriefing on our *Nutcracker* experience and discussing our plans for the holidays. Lisa invites us to join her and her husband, Gary, and son, Jake, for Christmas Day. We didn't expect this and are a little hesitant to intrude on someone's family Christmas Day dinner. Lisa, Gary and Jake have been such good friends, fully supporting us during my journey. They have become family. It just makes sense to say "yes!" Lisa's sister and her family will also be joining. We look forward to Christmas Day dinner with all of them.

Sunday, December 22

Our overnight stay at the Ritz Carlton is awesome! The bed is very comfortable. We spend the day meandering through the Christmas village around City Hall. Christmas decorations sparkle throughout the city. It's magical. We have a great time and then walk to the Sofitel hotel for lunch. We love the staff there, whom we see and visit with during lunch. Before leaving Philly, we stop at the best Italian deli, Di Bruno Bros., to pick up a few of our deli favorites!

Monday, December 23

We spend most of the day relaxing and running a few errands. We have really enjoyed having downtime from work. We end up watching a few Episodes of *Lost in Space*. Season 2 is definitely delivering!

We go to Wegmans to pick up our Christmas Eve dinner. Beforehand we go to see the latest Star Wars movie, *The Rise of Skywalker*. It's spectacular!

Tuesday, December 24

Scott and I spend our day relaxing and preparing our Christmas Eve dinner. We have a great day together and dinner is delicious! We bought a precooked, spiral-cut honey ham with scalloped potatoes and green beans. It is an easy meal to make with minimal clean-up. We open a nice bottle of Coppola Director's Cut Pinot Noir that we received from Gladys and Dan at our Celebration event. Dan is a biomarker marketing associate director at Merck. He and I work together developing biomarker tactics to support our biomarker strategy. I enjoy working with him, and he has become a good friend.

Wednesday, December 25

Christmas Day! It is a beautiful day. The temperature is around 40°F, and it's sunny. We have an invitation to Victoria and Steve's to share a Southern Christmas Day breakfast. As a gift, Scott and I bring a traditional *Panettone al Pistachio di Sicilia con Crema di Pistachio morbida da spalmare* (a delicious cake-like bread with pistachio cream frosting). Dolce & Gabbana makes this special-edition Sicilian delicacy in a beautiful tin container every year for Christmas.

Their home is awesome. Very tastefully done and extremely functional. One of the candles Victoria lit has a beautiful fragrance. It is the Aveda candle I gave her as a New Year's gift last year. Scott and I have a wonderful time celebrating Christmas morning with them. What a great way to start Christmas Day!

We have a few hours break in the afternoon before our dinner with Lisa and her family. We are able to take a nap, and I manage to fit in a horn practice session. My horn playing continues to show a dramatic improvement. I will definitely be recording the Beethoven Sonata in F Major, op. 17 soon.

We arrive at Lisa and Gary's at 5 PM to see the most magnificent Christmas tree we've ever seen in someone's home. It is at least fourteen feet high and seven feet wide, filled with ornaments from top to bottom and glistening with red lights. They went above and beyond with their Christmas decorating and dinner menu. There are cheeses, prosciutto and bacon-wrapped scallop appetizers—yummy! Gary labored for hours to prepare two premium filets. One is for those who like their meat rare and the other is for those who like their meat cooked. He seasoned and cooked each to perfection. Gary is definitely a savant chef.

Lisa's sister, Jen, along with her husband, Kevin, and their daughters, Lauren and Sofia, are also guests. We really enjoy our time with them. Earlier that day Jen had cut herself on a mandolin while making scalloped potatoes for our Christmas dinner. It's unfortunate, but we are able to find the humor and enjoy our time together. We listen to tracks in the background of Andrea Bocelli, Celine Dion and other artists performing holiday music. The ambiance is magical and desserts are plentiful. Lauren and Sofia made an awesome assortment of Christmas cookies, while

Gary provided several different types of delicious cheesecake. No one went home hungry.

This is one of the best Christmas Days ever!!!

Thursday, December 26

Scott and I spend the day relaxing, watching Netflix. We are so happy that *Lost in Space*, Season 2 was released on Netflix just before Christmas. Having grown up in the '60s, Scott and I have fond memories of the original TV series with the Robinson family. This new version provides an excellent modern-day update to the original series. It is pretty great, too.

Friday, December 27

Scott and I watch the last episode of *Lost in Space*. We've really enjoyed this Season 2. The transition from Season 1 is excellent, as Season 2 brings the story to a whole new level. Looks like there will be a lot of binge-watching this week.

Saturday, December 28

Scott and I meet Kyle and his wife, Sampty, for lunch at Basta Pasta in Skippack. It is so nice catching up and spending time with them. It was challenging to do so at our Celebration event with so many guests. We learn that they both play instruments: Sampty, the flute, and Kyle the trumpet. They both also like classical music and are very interested in attending a Philadelphia Orchestra concert with Scott and me. I mention that we are going to two concerts this spring. The first is at the beginning of March, when the Philadelphia Orchestra is performing Beethoven's Symphonies no. 5 and no. 6 as a tribute to Beethoven's 250th birthday celebration in 2020. There's also a performance the first week of

April of Symphonies 1 and 9. Beethoven's Symphony no. 9 is the one I hope they're able to attend.[41]

This morning, Scott and I packed our bags for an overnight stay at the new Four Seasons hotel in downtown Philadelphia, so after our lunch we're able to head directly there. At our Celebration of Life event, we received a very generous Four Seasons gift card from our friends and coworkers, Erica and Lauren, along with Gurinder, who works for one of Merck's marketing agencies. During our stay we'll meet Erica and her fiancée, Chris, for dinner here at the hotel's rooftop restaurant. Erica and Chris just became engaged on December 20! Between the dramatic improvement in my health and their engagement, there is lots to celebrate.

Scott and I arrive at the Four Seasons at 3:45 PM. Instantly, the service is what you would expect. We take the elevator from the lobby to check in on the sixtieth floor. The views are spectacular! Check-in is flawless, and we are accompanied to our room. On the way to our room, we discuss our dinner plans with the associate and realize that

---

[41.] *Music:*

Beethoven Symphony no. 5 in C Minor, op. 67 and Beethoven Symphony no. 6 in F Major, op. 68. Yannick Nézet-Séguin and the Philadelphia Orchestra BeethovenNow Concert Series, March 2020 performance (YouTube video, 1:26:35). Symphony no. 5 begins at minute 10:37. It is proceeded by the opening performance of Habibi's "Jeder Baum spricht." Posted by the Philadelphia Orchestra, March 14, 2020; accessed November 2020. *https://www.youtube.com/watch?v=zKWYX5ohadQ*

Beethoven, Symphony No. 1 in C Major, op 21. Sir Georg Solti conducting the Chicago Symphony Orchestra (YouTube video, 31:01). Posted by Ahmed Barod on December 4, 2012; posted by Louis Cesarini February 4, 2021. *https://www.youtube.com/watch?v=Pj2neof3MIs*

Beethoven Symphony no. 9 in D Minor, op. 125 "Choral." The Mormon Tabernacle Choir, Eugene Ormandy and the Philadelphia Orchestra (YouTube video, 1:08:14). Minute 44:18 marks the opening of the fourth and final movement. Posted by soy ink, August 24, 2017; accessed September 2020. *https://www.youtube.com/watch?v=eb_vUFxgtxM*

the restaurant we want to dine at is Jean-Georges on the fifty-ninth floor, rather than Vernick Fish, which is located on the ground floor. The associate immediately offers to see if they can change our reservation. Within minutes after seeing us to our room, we receive a call letting us know this is done. Needless to say, we are thrilled. Erica and Chris meet us at 7 PM, and we share a bottle of Veuve Clicquot between us. It's been months since I've had any alcohol, so one glass does it for me! Our dinner at Jean-Georges is absolutely superb! Our seating provides a spectacular 270-degree view of the city of Philadelphia. We enjoy a fabulous time with Erica and Chris.

....

Sunday, December 29

This morning we head to the indoor heated pool. It's on a high floor with a beautiful view of the city. The water temperature is perfect, and the views are incredible! We settle in once we're back home and watch an episode of *The Big Bang Theory*. This is the episode (no. 13 from Season 5) where Leonard and Penny begin dating again. In an attempt to lessen the pressure, Leonard uses a computer analogy, "2.0," to brand their renewed relationship. You guessed it; this is where the idea to brand myself "Louis 2.0" came from.

This evening, I begin recording my performance of the Beethoven Horn Sonata in F Major, op. 17. It goes very well. I record all three movements with a second recording of movements one and two. Movement three needs a little work still, so I'll look to re-record that movement tomorrow. I am very pleased with how the recordings turned out. Although I could live with these recordings, I know I can do better.

After my recording session, I break down in Scott's arms filled with the emotion of how well the session went. This is a lifetime's dream come true. I am the horn player I've always dreamed of being. The best part about this is that I have been able to achieve this despite my current disease progression with stage 4 lung cancer. Take that, cancer!

Monday, December 30

It's hard to believe that 2019 is almost over. Certainly, though bittersweet, it has been one of our best years. Scott and I continue to focus on the good we have versus my cancer. We say that 10 percent of a challenge is what it is. The other 90 percent is what you do and how you choose to respond. We choose staying positive and focusing on solutions.

Tuesday, December 31

Scott and I are looking forward to bringing in the new year tonight. As part of our celebration, we're preparing a special New Year's Eve dinner: my mom's homemade spaghetti sauce and meatballs. It's been simmering all day, filling up the house with wonderful aromas. Mary Lou Cesarini, your love lives in my heart and dreams always.

Mary Lou's Homemade
Spaghetti Sauce & Meatballs

I am including this recipe as a tribute to my mom, Mary Lou. I'm not sure if she created this recipe herself or if it was passed down. Mom's homemade sauce, along with her meatball recipe, is always at the top of Scott's and my list of the dinners we create to celebrate birthdays, anniversaries, holidays and any other special event we can think of as an excuse to make mom's sauce. Throughout the years, we have experimented with mom's recipe. The version here uses her recipe as the base, and we tailor it to make it our own. We hope you enjoy it as much as we do.

To make the sauce: We use a 9-quart Le Creuset, or any large saucepot works. Be sure to keep the gas flame or electric heat on the lowest setting throughout the entire cooking process. Cooking slow helps prevent the sauce from burning, and the low heat allows the sauce to slowly gel with the spices. Scott and I often have had my mom's sauce cooking for hours, from morning to early evening.

The amounts of ingredients used will allow you to make enough sauce so that you have plenty left over for next time—more on the importance of that later. To begin, with the heat on low, add 2 circles of your favorite olive oil to the bottom of your saucepot. Add 2 tablespoons chopped garlic. Combine 6 ripe Roma wedged tomatoes and 18 ounces of tomato paste with about 16 ounces of water, depending how thick you like your sauce. Chop fresh oregano, thyme, parsley, basil and add them to the pot along with salt and pepper to taste.

Now you're ready to add the main "secret" ingredient: a sweet onion with a ribbon of whole cloves. Slice the top and bottom portions of an onion about halfway through. Gently peel away a layer of onion. Insert whole cloves, like winding a ribbon, centered in the middle and around the sides of the onion, keeping about an eighth of an inch distance between each clove until it completes the circle. One ring of whole cloves is all that's needed. Place the onion with its ribbon of cloves in the middle of the sauce. As it cooks, it will create an aroma like nothing you've ever experienced!

Once the sauce and its ingredients have cooked for about 2 hours at low heat, add a combination of sweet and hot Italian sausage. We've had the best results with Johnsonville sausage, as it always is very tender as it cooks slowly with the sauce. Even though we're adding the raw sausage links directly to the sauce, you can keep the heat on the lowest setting so as to continue the slow cooking process. The flavors of the sausage blend with the sauce as it cooks. After a few hours, you'll want to remove the onion and cloves. We always wait until the onion is so tender that it almost falls apart before removing it from the sauce.

To make the meatballs: While the sauce is cooking, prepare the meatballs. In a large bowl, add equal parts of ground beef, ground pork and ground veal, about 1 pound of each. You can replace the meat with appropriate vegan-friendly ingredients or turkey if desired. Add the ground meat all together in the bowl, along with 2 eggs, and the same spices used for the sauce: fresh oregano, thyme, parsley, basil, and salt and pepper to taste. Have ready 3 slices of stale bread, one for each pound of meat. Break apart the bread into small pieces, like large bread crumbs and add them to the bowl. Add 1 cup of Parmigiano Reggiano along with 2 tablespoons of chopped garlic. Include 1 large sweet onion, chopped into small pieces. Using clean, bare hands (this is how the Italians do it), mix all of these ingredients together. Add about ⅔ cup 2% milk a little bit at a time as you mush, until you've reached the point where there is medium density to the mixture. It will feel very mushy using your bare hands, but that's what makes it fun! As all of the ingredients are combined, you'll begin to feel that you're at the point when meatballs can take shape. We make our meatballs pretty large, usually the size of baseballs. You'll end up with 8 or 9 meatballs.

When the sausages are tender, remove them from the sauce so as to make room for the meatballs. Allow your cooked sausages to cool before placing them in a covered bowl. (You'll want to reheat the sausage right before you boil your pasta so that everything is warm and ready to go when your pasta is done.)

Now it's time to add the handmade raw meatballs to the sauce. As with the sausages, keep the heat low so the meatballs can cook slowly. The additional flavors of the meatballs will add to the already existing taste. Adding the meatballs raw will result in tender, tasty meatballs that aren't overcooked. After about 6 hours, when the sauce is smooth to taste with all ingredients blended, versus bold and in your face, it will be ready to serve. You could shut off the heat anytime during the 6-hour time period; just be sure the lid is on tight so the sauce can continue to reduce. Shortly before serving, reheat the sausages by stirring them back into the sauce. We use Tagliatelle for our pasta to serve with the sauce and sometimes we include a side dish of mixed vegetables like cut zucchini and carrots.

Certainly, this dish is not something that takes a short amount of time. My mom always began cooking her sauce first thing Sunday morning, continuing on through the rest of the day until dinnertime at 6 PM. Smelling her delicious sauce cooking on the stove all day is one of my cherished childhood memories of my mom, one that I hold deeply in my heart. I am happy to share it with you!

The secret of the leftover sauce: One time, on a trip to a champagne cellar in Reims, France, Scott and I learned through a tour why high-end champagnes, like the yellow label of Veuve Clicquot, don't have a vintage year on the bottle. The reason is that the champagne maker uses a portion of each year's yield to create the next year's champagne. This makes for a consistent-tasting champagne from year to year. Since the champagne is a blend of multiple years, the champagne maker is unable to place a specific vintage year on the bottle.

Scott and I use this same methodology to great effect with mom's sauce. Mom's sauce and meatballs can be frozen. (Sausage doesn't freeze well.) Each time we make the sauce, before adding the meat, we save and freeze a portion of the sauce for next time. Just be sure to take it out of the freezer the night before and place it in the refrigerator to thaw overnight. This thawed portion of sauce is what you'll start cooking with first as you begin to add the ingredients I mention to make a new sauce. Throughout the years, Scott and I have enjoyed continuing my mom's spaghetti sauce and meatball legacy. We used to find that each time we made the sauce, it tasted a little different than it did before. This "champagne" process of preserving a frozen portion eliminates any inconsistencies each time the sauce is made.

I feel like I'm in the "sweet spot" with my horn playing lately. I'm not sure what's on the road ahead, so it is important for me to capture this time now and finish recording Beethoven's Sonata in F Major, op. 17 as soon as possible.

I did it! It goes even better than yesterday. This is the recording I will put on YouTube. What a great way to finish the year! I am very proud of this achievement. Tears of joy run down my face as

I think about all that I'm going through: thirteen brain metastases, the return of the lesion on my spine combined with all the medication I'm on. I'm so happy to be putting music into the world.

Our New Year's Eve Italian dinner is superb! The sauce and meatballs are as wonderful as ever. We have a glass of 2012 Oro Ducale Chianti with dinner. It goes very well with our meal. We started the evening with a glass of 1999 Dom Perignon. We've been saving the bottle especially for tonight. After all, what's New Year's Eve without a glass of champagne? It tasted quite good for a twenty-year-old champagne. We'll save the rest so as not to overdo it.

Scott and I spend our evening reminiscing about all that we've been through this year and wonder about what the new year will bring. During one of our toasts, Scott looks me in the eye and says he is happy I am here. This says it all. I say, "I'm happy I'm here," as tears stream down my cheeks. We focus on how grateful we are to have each other, for all we have, versus what we don't have. There's a lot to be thankful for, lots to celebrate.

We watch a few traditional New Year's Eve celebrations around the world as midnight rings in the new year. There is a silent moment as Scott and I again look into each other's eyes. We know what the other is thinking, but neither one of us says a word. We kiss and give each other a big hug. It's sleep time. Happy New Year, everyone!

January 2020

Wednesday, January 1

Happy 2020!!! We are having a great day! We watch part of the Mummers Parade, a Philadelphia must, along with the Rose Parade live from Pasadena, California. We especially love the Rose Parade based on having lived in Southern California for many years. Scott lived there one year before meeting me, and I lived there five years before meeting him in 1993. You can take the boys out of So Cal, but you can't take the So Cal out of the boys!

....

Thursday, January 2

I went to the office today. It is the first time I've actually gone in since before our November Celebration event. Since my setback, we thought it best that I focus on my health, eliminate any undue stress and work from home for the balance of 2019. That was a good decision.

It is quiet in the office. Only the diehards are here. It's great seeing my coworkers, especially those who attended our Celebration event.

In the evening Scott and I watch a new movie, *Marriage Story* with Scarlett Johansson and Adam Driver. I won't give away too many spoilers, but essentially it's a story of a couple going through a divorce. Near the beginning, their marriage counselor recommends that they each write about why they married. The purpose of this is to have a reminder of the good that brought them together as they maneuver through the separation/divorce process.

I decide this is a good opportunity to write the same about Scott. When Scott and I met on November 20, 1993, I instantly knew he was the one.

Scott is a happy person. He is very positive and always smiles, even during challenging times. He has beautiful hazel eyes (just like my mom had). They sparkle ever so beautifully. Scott loves animals. He is gentle and very caring. He is a healer. Scott is tender. He is always willing to help others. He is a very hard worker, always looking to improve his skills in order to deliver excellence to his customers. He loves me more than anyone ever has. He shows this through his actions in addition to his words. Scott is very patient. He is the best kisser! My life with Scott has been a fairy tale. Our journey together since my diagnosis of stage 4 lung cancer has only strengthened our bond. I am the luckiest guy in the world to have such a loving, dedicated, caring husband!!!

Friday, January 3

I work from home and have a productive day. Work email is very quiet. Many colleagues extended their holiday break to include this week. Good for them. I don't mind working given the two-week Orient Express trip we're taking in April. We're counting the days!

I continue to feel great! No pain, no fatigue, no nausea, no GI problems, no problems sleeping with 100 percent energy level. I have to imagine that my brain metastases are gone or nearly gone. Monday's scan will determine that. This is our hope. If history is an indicator, my scans have always directly reflected how I feel.

Saturday, January 4

Scott and I plan to post my Beethoven Sonata in F Major, op. 17 to YouTube tomorrow. We are so excited! What a great way to end 2019 and start the new year 2020!

We have a wonderful lunch get-together with our friends Dan and Gladys, and in the evening we meet Victoria and Steve for dinner at Firebirds in Providence Town Center, Collegeville. Dinner lasts three hours as we revisit what we all did over the holidays. Victoria and Steve spent New Year's Eve at the Kimmel Center, ringing in the new year with the Philadelphia Orchestra. They share with us that Strauss was flowing with echoes of the "Blue Danube" filling the concert hall. Scott and I are thrilled to hear how they celebrated the coming of the new year as a newly married couple.

After dinner, we are standing outside before leaving. I share with Victoria and Steve something I had shared with Scott earlier at home before we left for dinner. I say that although the news of my stage 4 lung cancer was tragic this past year, I can't remember being happier than I am now. My perspective on life has changed. Every day is truly a gift. Scott and I are so very happy that my quality of life has improved back to 100 percent. Every day we wake up and look at each other in amazement as we start another day. We are so grateful.

Victoria and Steve look at me in astonishment with tears welling up in their eyes. We all give each other a big hug and say goodnight.

....

Sunday, January 5

Scott and I spend most of the afternoon posting my Beethoven Sonata in F Major, op. 17 for Horn and Piano to YouTube. It isn't easy. There are lots of intricacies with YouTube that neither one of us realized beforehand. But we did it! This recording of Beethoven's Horn Sonata in F Major, op. 17 is a tribute to Ludwig van Beethoven's 250th birthday. Beethoven was born on or about December 16, 1770, in Bonn, Germany. The year 2020 marks the 250th year celebration of his birth. Here is my YouTube Introduction:

> This December 31, 2019, recording is performed by Louis Vincent Cesarini (Louis 2.0) accompanied by his Yamaha Disklavier. It is dedicated to my husband, Scott; my horn teacher, Jack McCammon; Jen Montone; the Curtis Institute of Music Summerfest students, alumni, faculty and staff; Reimund Pankratz and the entire staff at Gebr. Alexander Horns, Mainz, Germany; and all our dear friends and coworkers. Without your support, this recording would not have been possible.
>
> Ludwig van Beethoven composed his Horn Sonata in F Major, op. 17 in 1800 for the virtuoso horn player Giovanni Punto. It was premiered with Punto as the soloist, accompanied on the piano by Beethoven himself in Vienna on April 18, 1800.

Recording Beethoven's Horn Sonata in F major, op. 17 is a lifelong dream. One I am very proud to have achieved.[42]

....

Monday, January 6

We head to the Radnor Penn Medicine Radiology Center for my MRI of the brain with and without contrast scheduled for today. I receive a call early this morning from Bailey, a radiology administrative assistant, with whom I spoke late Friday. Bailey says she will reach out to our insurance company first thing this morning to get prior authorization approval for my MRI with contrast. I shared with Bailey on Friday that all my MRIs have been with and without contrast so there should not be any issue receiving insurance approval. As promised, Bailey calls shortly after 9 AM to confirm that the prior authorization has been approved with contrast and asks if we can show up at 11 AM, which is not a problem. The staff at Penn Medicine is consistently great.

Now that Dr. Langer is my primary oncologist, all of my scans and MRIs moving forward will be through Penn Medicine. My previous MRIs and CT scans were completed at Abington-Jefferson locations when Dr. CO was my primary oncologist. Unfortunately, Radnor Penn Medicine Radiology doesn't have the capability to use headphones and pipe in music like Abington-Jefferson. This is due to the differences in the MRI machines. So, in order to distract myself, I play the Beethoven Horn Sonata over and over in my head. It works! I can practically see the music in front of me as my eyes are closed inside the MRI machine. I didn't realize I had most of it memorized until now. It makes for a very positive MRI

[42.] *Music:* Beethoven: Sonata in F Major, op. 17 for Horn and Piano. Louis V. Cesarini (Louis 2.0), French horn; piano, Yamaha Disklavier. YouTube video playlist: update posted by Louis Cesarini, July 11, 2020. *https://www.youtube.com/ playlist?list=PLD3OTBbtvFjmyAorvSgeXVBBIO7gVpVRt*

experience. Anyone who has had an MRI knows distracting yourself in some way is hands down better than actively listening to what sounds like a bunch of hammers clunking around in a dryer for thirty minutes.

Back at home, I play the Mozart Concerto Rondo, K371, a piece I haven't played in probably thirty years. I have a memory of playing it during a practice session when I was visiting my mom years ago. Mom liked how it bounces around. It is a lovely memory of my mother that I cherish. We have the MIDI disk with the accompaniment, so I am able to play it on our Yamaha Disklavier. It goes pretty fast, so you just have to jump in.

§

I receive a late-night text from Jack with feedback on my YouTube recording:

> Bravo bravo!!!! Amazing job! Wow, I am so impressed, such great work! Sorry for the later reply, spending the evening with my parents before I head back to Philly tomorrow morning! I loved your commitment and drive. The second movement was delicate and sweet. Beautiful! And the third movement was energetic and buoyant. I loved it! Are you feeling up to starting lessons again? Will you use this for Summerfest? Let me know! Very exciting, Louis 2.0!!!!!

I read Jack's text and feel so happy to be living this moment.

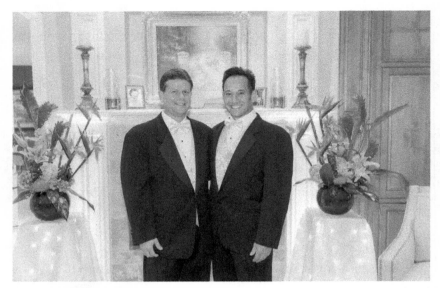

Our Wedding Day, November 20, 2015

Part IV
Believe

Movement 4
Presto: Allegro assai[43]

*The final movement of Beethoven's 9th Symphony
contains the famous theme "Ode to Joy." "Allegro"
is Italian for joyful; "assai" is defined as very. You
can hear echoes of melodies from previous movements. In this
last movement, it all comes together with a jubilant theme
and triumphant ending!*

[43.] *Music:* Beethoven: Symphony no. 9 in D Minor, op. 125 "Choral." The
Mormon Tabernacle Choir, Eugene Ormandy and the Philadelphia Orchestra
(YouTube video, 1:08:14). Minute 44:18 marks the opening of the fourth and
final movement. Posted by soy ink, August 24, 2017; accessed September 2020.
https://www.youtube.com/watch?v=eb_vUFxgtxM

Beethoven's 9th Symphony shattered conventional thinking of how the structure of a symphony should be. He added a chorus and four solo singers in a fourth movement that in duration alone could be the same as a full symphony. Symphony no. 9 has inspired me throughout my life. It's beautiful and very powerful. I think about the struggles Beethoven experienced during his lifetime. Can you imagine writing this symphony being totally deaf? What Beethoven couldn't hear with his ears, he heard in his mind and felt in his heart—this is what he shares with us.

The musical composition is genius: a celebration of sound, various melodies with intense, powerful dynamics. It's among the best symphonies ever written, over 196 years later. If Beethoven were alive today, I hope he would be proud to know I consider his 9th Symphony a masterpiece and a depiction of my journey with lung cancer. The music defines me letting go, sharing what's in my soul and the totality of my lung cancer journey with the world.

I don't know how my battle against lung cancer will end up playing itself out, but I do believe I've lived a lifetime of many dreams come true. I am reminded of the words Dr. Langer shared with us at our Celebration of Life, Love and Friendship event back in November: "By hook or by crook, we'll get there." I'm not a religious person, but I am very spiritual. I've always had a sixth sense about things, though one could argue if it were any good I would have "seen" my lung cancer way back when it first started. Oh, well. What I do see in my rearview mirror is my mother standing on the front porch waving goodbye to me as I left for California. This would be the last time I would see her. I see Scott, the love of my life, whom I consider a gift from my mom who never wanted me to grow old alone. I see the wonderful life I've lived so far. So many wonderful memories! There is nothing I would change. I have no regrets. My life was written just the way it was supposed to be. Whether I have months or years left to my life, I know my days ahead will be equally wonderful. For anyone on a similar journey, the reward is big; we just have to believe.

January 2020

··

Tuesday, January 7

Scott and I wake up feeling hopeful that my brain metastases are gone. We can't imagine anything other than positive results given how good I feel and also the fact I just made the best French horn recording of my life on YouTube with the Beethoven Sonata for Horn and Piano in F Major, op. 17. How could I have had the bandwidth capability to concentrate with tumors lurking around in my brain?

I work from home today, as I did yesterday, due to my medical appointments. I am looking forward to going back into the office tomorrow for the rest of the week. It will be good to see everyone.

This morning, my good friend and coworker James calls me to catch up on his way into work. I always enjoy my conversations with James. He's very supportive. He and his wife, Pam, and their child, Luca, drove down to Charleston to spend the holidays with family. Although it was hectic with all the driving, they enjoyed their time away.

Another good friend and coworker, Kristen, and I are looking to schedule a visit with her husband, Michael, and their daughter, Sabrina. We arrange to meet for lunch on January 31. Scott and I look forward to our time with them.

Scott and I are looking to leave at 12:45 PM for our 1:45 PM appointment with Dr. Langer. We are having chicken soup for lunch and saving room for a delicious hot slice of pizza from the ground-level bistro at Penn Medicine. It's always a hectic day going to this appointment in downtown Philadelphia between street traffic and the traffic of patients coming and going into the cancer center. It's a well-oiled machine though. Aside from the long wait to get your car back from valet parking, it is a flawless process. This time Scott is going to drop me off and then park the car so we don't have to wait an extra hour for valet after our appointment.

Today we will be reviewing my MRI brain scan results with Dr. Langer. The Flaura registration study for Tagrisso recommends that you do the first MRI of the brain at six weeks from the time you start. With the identification of thirteen brain metastases, there's no time to wait that long; we're doing it at four weeks. We need to be proactive just in case. Given that I've been a hyper-responder and that I'm feeling good, Scott and I are holding strong with our optimism.

I was dubbed a "hyper-responder" by my friends Victoria and Lisa. They both have shared, during various moments of my treatment, that I respond quickly to any treatment I receive. Victoria shared with me, back when I was going through my radiation treatments, that she's never met anyone who is as in tune with their body as I am.

§

Drum roll, please! We have news. As Scott and I are waiting for Dr. Langer, his fellow, whom I'll refer to as Dr. N, comes in to ask if we have seen the results from my brain MRI. We say no, and Dr. N proceeds to share that I had a "remarkable response" to Tagrisso. My brain mets are gone! All thirteen of them. There are faint remnants of the largest one that was 1.5 cm. I jump up and put my arms in the air and scream with joy. Then I burst into tears.

I have my life back!!!

I've never before cried happy tears so intensely. I sit back with amazement to digest the news. It is an unbelievable moment.

Dr. Langer comes in about thirty minutes later with a big smile on his face. He pulls up the imaging to review my November brain MRI alongside this current one. It is an incredible moment as we look and compare both MRIs. It is literally night and day as he compares both images. I really was in trouble with thirteen tumors in my brain, mostly small. The large 1.5-cm tumor was most concerning and the reason why I was on 4 mg of dexamethasone daily. Now the lesions have been obliterated, and it is difficult to find and see any definitive image of the big lesion. What we do see is very small. It looks like a planet in *Star Wars* that was hit by a laser and obliterated into pieces. Dr. Langer says I can reduce my dexamethasone to 2 mg daily, taken morning and evening, and I get to do this immediately—yeah!

All of this is happening after only thirty days of taking 80 mg of Tagrisso once a day. The next steps will be a CT scan with contrast and an MRI of my spine.

I continue to be in a surreal cloud of exuberance as we finish our time with Dr. Langer and then move over to the infusion center, right next to where Dr. Langer's patient rooms are located. Today I will be getting Xgeva, an injectable drug that helps increase bone density. This is to promote new bone growth, including in my spine, from any bone deterioration caused by cancer lesions. It's good to have my future back. Cancer is losing this battle.

It's been quite the process. As a stage 4 lung cancer patient, I had to go through a prior authorization process to get Xgeva approved. When I started my lung cancer journey last May, prior to my first Keytruda Combo infusion, my community oncologist tried to get Xgeva approved by my insurance company. Xgeva is delivered by a single subcutaneous injection to the arm, once every four weeks. Due to the high cost, it was denied by my insurance for first-line treatment. I needed to take Zometa first and fail it before Xgeva could be approved. Zometa also promotes bone growth, but it's given via IV every six weeks versus a subcutaneous shot.

When my spine bone lesion returned, based on my November CT scan, this confirmed that Zometa had failed. Since I transitioned to Dr. Langer at Penn Medicine in early December, he and I decided to make the case for Xgeva moving forward. Before this could happen, I had to call my community oncologist's nurse, ask her to confirm with the doctor that I had failed Zometa and document this in my Abington-Jefferson patient information. I then had to call Dr. CO's prior authorization insurance reimbursement manager, Barb, to ask her to physically call my insurance company to let them know I had failed Zometa. I received a call from Barb when this was done.

Then I had to call Penn Medicine to speak with Dr. Langer's nurse. I needed to help them connect the dots so I could receive Xgeva on my next visit. Zometa had formally failed, and a process needed to occur with my insurance company so that Xgeva could be approved. Dr. Langer's nurse captured this information in my patient record. I then received a call from the Penn Medicine prior authorization point person, who confirmed that they had all the documentation and insurance approvals needed for me to begin Xgeva. I would receive it during my appointment today with Dr. Langer. All of this occurred at the end of December. It was an arduous process, but well worth the time to ensure I would receive Xgeva.

The prior authorization process may sound familiar to you. It's crazy! Don't assume your doctor's office, i.e., healthcare provider, is aware of any changes to your insurance and/or medications. Treatments can be withheld if our insurance companies aren't aligned with changes. Every procedure, scan or MRI needs a prior authorization approval. However exhausting, patients or caregivers have to communicate with all parties to facilitate connecting the dots on necessary approvals. As Scott and I were waiting to get my Xgeva injection, a woman was there, in a wheelchair. She looked frail, tired and wore a headwrap. The type you see cancer patients wear when they are losing their hair. Apparently, she had recently changed her insurance from what she had in 2019 to new insurance in 2020 based on the open conversation her caretakers were having with the medical assistants checking them in. By the way the conversation went, it seemed like they were waiting most of the day for their sister, the person in the wheelchair, to get treatment. I believe that she may have been a lung cancer patient since we were on the floor and in the area where Dr. Langer and other lung oncologists are located.

It was heart-wrenching seeing her diminished performance status and hearing her caretakers explain the change of insurance to the medical assistant receptionist. Apparently, they had communicated the information on the new insurance to Penn Medicine prior to arriving at the cancer center for treatment. It sounded identical to the prior authorization process I had just gone through, but with a disconnect. The patient and her caregivers did not know what they didn't know, and the step about letting their oncologist's staff know about the change in insurance was missed. Her physician's prior authorization administrator with Penn Medicine was most likely unaware of the change in insurance companies ahead of their treatment visit. It is my understanding that no patient can receive treatment unless the oncology cancer center can confirm payment. Medical providers want to make sure they are going to be reimbursed for any medications a patient receives *before* they will give it to a patient. If the cancer doesn't beat us up, the insurance process will. It shouldn't be this way, especially for cancer patients.

Tears streamed down my face as I looked at the patient and listened to the passionate pleas from the siblings to approve their sister's chemotherapy treatment. That could have been me if I didn't know what I know. What I was witnessing is more the rule than not in our current healthcare system. I don't know what the outcome was, but I am sad to think that the change in the patient's healthcare insurance caused the prior authorization process to be incomplete. Because of this, it is unlikely that this cancer patient received treatment that day. I hope I'm wrong. It was 5 PM, the end of the day, and by the way she looked, she needed this treatment to help her stay alive.

This is but one real-world example of how complicated our healthcare process can be. The prior authorization process gives your health insurance company a chance to review how necessary a certain treatment is based on your medical condition. Be sure to check with your doctor on any prior authorizations needed when any medications, tests or procedures are being considered for you. Often, the physician may already know what medications are or are not covered based on your insurance. Either way, be sure to ask, don't assume.

Remember that WE, as patients, have so much power. More than we may realize. Use that power and advocate for yourself as you navigate the multilayered healthcare system.

Wednesday, January 8

I go into the office today. Everyone is back from the holiday break. I see many coworkers that I haven't seen since our November celebration event. It's so good seeing everyone!

Scott and I continue to discuss the great news from yesterday and share how happy we are to be back to this point. Certainly, we knew it had to be good news based on how good I've been feeling along with the dramatic improvement in my horn playing. I continue to practice my horn at night to refine the Mozart Horn Concerto #3 in E-flat Major. This is the next piece I'm looking to record and post online.

Thursday, January 9

I continue to feel well and go into the office. There is no disconnect between how I feel and those positive brain MRI results. I have a few meetings and need to prepare for my upcoming marketing interviews. During the holidays, I applied for two internal positions; both are in marketing.

Friday, January 10

Today I go into the office for a meeting that lasts from 9 AM until 2 PM. I stay another hour so Lisa and I can catch up. Scott and I bought a Nutcracker tree ornament just after Christmas. We thought of Lisa and her family's big beautiful Christmas tree. The ornament perfectly captures our time with them during the holidays.

I always listen to the classical music station WRTI when I am in the car. On the way into the office this morning, literally minutes after I pull out of our driveway, the radio announcer comes on and says: "Next we're going to hear the only piece written by Beethoven for horn."

I freeze, knowing that his Sonata in F Major, op. 17 is the only piece Beethoven ever wrote for horn. The announcer echoes my thoughts:

Beethoven wrote a single piece for horn and piano. His Sonata in F Major was written in 1800 for a friend of his who played horn, Giovanni Punto. This piece was so challenging to play that it remained un-played by any other horn player for over a year after it premiered in 1800 with Punto performing while Beethoven himself played the piano accompaniment. Given that a year had gone by, Beethoven wrote another version of this Sonata for cello.

I listen in amazement at the extreme coincidence, all the while knowing I continue to be reminded that there is no such thing as a coincidence. All that I've experienced in life has brought me to this point. This musical example is just one more piece of the puzzle.

Saturday, January 11

It's a beautiful 60°F sunny day! We'll take that for mid-January any day. Scott and I enjoy a nice ham-and-egg croissant. We bought some specialty sandwiches from Williams-Sonoma just before the holidays and have been enjoying them for breakfast since.

I have a good thirty-minute warm-up on my horn in preparation for my noon lesson with Jack. Today's lesson is the best one ever. I know I may have said that before, but they truly are getting better! We play up and down several octaves of scales as a warm-up refresher. At my request, we go up a half step from F to high C. This is the first time Jack has heard me play above a G. It feels great. I have the muscle strength in my embouchure now that helps my endurance. All I need is more air to support my sound. It's not easy, but I power through it and keep practicing. I know what it feels like; now I just need to keep doing it so I can easily maneuver throughout all the registers covered by the French horn. I know it's right when my lips feel like they are floating on the mouthpiece. This is when the real fun of playing the French horn begins.

I tell Jack about what I heard on the radio yesterday. He wasn't aware that there was a cello version and is surprised at the coincidence of hearing it right after I posted my own recording.

After my lesson, Scott and I stop at Di Bruno's deli. We have lunch and pick up chicken marsala to have for dinner tonight. We have a 2008 Lewis Reserve Chardonnay that Scott found when he was organizing our wine collection over the holidays. Dinner is great, and the wine makes for a perfect pairing. It is so nice being outside tonight. The temperature is still 60°F at 7 PM. We watch a couple 2Cello music videos. It is magical.

Sunday, January 12

Scott is taking online courses as part of maintaining his PMP certification. He came across this analogy that is taken from *Game of Thrones*: "Every bruise is a lesson, and every lesson makes us stronger." The character Arya Stark, played by Maisie Williams, says this, and I think it's highly relevant to my journey. Scott and I are huge *GOT* fans!

Scott and I go for a 2.5-mile walk on the Perkiomen Trail today. The sun is nice and warm like yesterday. The temperature reaches 64°F. Later we are able to connect on a FaceTime call with Caro and Dano! It has been a while since we last spoke. They have been celebrating Caro's birthday, which was January 2.

She loves sweets and spends the entire month of January eating cakes and sweet things. You'd never know to look at her as she is about ninety-five pounds soaking wet! Dano was in the process of making a coconut cake with coconut pudding filling between two layers. Doesn't that sound yummy?

I play through the Beethoven Horn Sonata in F Major, op. 17 tonight to review a few areas. I want to be sure to capture Jack's feedback. My timing and interpretation are noticeably better.

Monday, January 13

I wake up feeling great! I was initially going to work from home but based on how well I feel, I decide to go into the office. Being in-person at meetings is so much more beneficial to understanding meeting topics and dynamics than calling in. Plus, it's great to see everyone.

I continue to practice my horn at night. Each session is consistent with the last. I am zipping through my warm-up scales in all octaves, like a pro. I'm not overextending my embouchure. I'm letting the air move me through each note as my ability to support and control continues to dramatically improve. I continue to have that floating feeling on the mouthpiece. This assures me that I'm on the right track.

Tuesday, January 14

I have an eye appointment this morning at 8:30 AM. Scott has meetings so I drive myself there. This is a follow-up appointment from my last exam six months ago. I share my current progress with Tagrisso with Dr. O (as I'll call him), and he is thrilled to hear this news. He says I look great: "alert and vibrant." Wow! I'm always so tough on myself. This is just what I need to hear.

I receive a glowing check-up on my eyes. I thank Dr. O as I share my most recent scare with brain metastasis and tell him how much I value my vision. In hindsight, no pun intended, I can recall reading wrong notes around the same time I had my setback. Certainly, this could be related to the cognitive effects of having thirteen brain lesions. I'm so happy they are gone! I'm definitely not hitting many wrong notes now.

Each day this week, I continue to feel better. I started taking an iron supplement over the weekend since my red blood cells have consistently been at the low end of the scale. I believe this is working as I have more energy and have been able to go into the office daily.

....

Friday, January 17

I am so happy to be feeling good! I am not experiencing any fatigue, particularly in the afternoon, around 2 PM, as I did when I was on Keytruda Combo every three weeks. Now each day I feel "normal." My energy level is close to 100 percent. Not sure how this is going to pan out with the amount of cancer still in me, but I'll know after my February 3 full CT scan. My primary lesion was 3 × 3 cm last time. I'm hoping it's 1 × 1 cm or less this time, if not gone, and that all other metastases, lymph nodes and lesions correspond in size.

....

Saturday, January 18

Scott and I spend most of the day cleaning the house. This includes dusting furniture and mopping our large floor in the living room, dining room, laundry room, hallway, kitchen, dinette area and family room. We divide and conquer. It takes some time and is a lot of work, but that's okay because I have lots of energy today! The house looks great!

We make a homemade dinner. Scott puts together slices of squash, broccoli florets, Roma tomatoes, mushrooms and sliced chicken breast to make a primavera that includes olive oil garlic, shallots and red pepper flakes. We add orecchiette pasta and Locatelli cheese, which gives it that special zing. We open a bottle of Santa Margherita Pinot Grigio, which I haven't tasted in months. It is wonderful!

As a homage to our beloved Dalmatians, Casper, Tiffany and Lance, we watch the original *The Sound of Music*. We said good-bye to Casper and Tiffany fourteen years ago today, and to Lance, ten years ago today. Yes, the same day, four years apart. It just worked out that way. Losing our Dalmatians, Scott's mom on December 7, 2007, and my dad on November 28, 2014, was difficult. The loss of our loved ones during the holidays is the single-most reason we stopped decorating our home for Christmas and instead began traveling to warm places. We had our fill of having that horrible pit feeling in our stomachs during the holidays. Most recently, after thirty-two years, we lost our dear cockatoo, Amadeus, on June 6, 2018.

This year, that seems to have changed, especially after this Christmas with all the wonderful moments Scott and I shared celebrating my improved health, spending Christmas Day with Victoria, Steve, Lisa, Gary, Jake and Lisa's sister and her family. We just might be decorating our home for Christmas next year!

Sunday, January 19

Today I wake up feeling fuzzy and fatigued. I hadn't felt like this since I started Tagrisso. Not sure why I'm feeling this way. Maybe because I started reducing my dexamethasone on Friday, and it's been two days now. My body might be adjusting as it transitions off dexamethasone. Dr. Langer's nurse practioner, Susie, mentioned this might occur during my mid-December appointment with her. I was taking dexamethasone to reduce the inflammation in my brain and spine caused by the lesions. Dexamethasone is significantly more potent than prednisolone. Considering its potency, how I'm feeling is most likely due to my body transitioning off dexamethasone. Luckily, I am home, off from work, and have a pretty easy day. We're meeting our friends Lucy and Jon for lunch, but that is literally down the street, five minutes from our home at Basta Pasta. Scott and I last saw them in November at our Celebration of Life, Love and Friendship event. We enjoy our time together and have a wonderful visit.

Monday, January 20

I feel much better today, back to my usual self. I have plenty of energy and feel good. I'm not sure what all that was about yesterday. I am off work today. We have a company holiday in commemoration of Martin Luther King Jr. Day. It is great spending the day at home with Scott, who actually does not have the day off. I continue to prepare for my upcoming marketing interviews and then run some errands. I go to the AT&T store to replace my screen protector on my new iPhone. My phone fell out of my jacket pocket last weekend when Scott and I were getting out of the car to take a walk on the Perkiomen Trail. Thank goodness I had a screen protector. It got pretty marked up in the left corner. My new iPhone screen protector is better (and more expensive) than the one I had. Hopefully, I won't be dropping my phone any more, but then again, that's why we have screen protectors.

Tuesday, January 21

I feel good today. I continue to go into the office to work, versus working from home. My energy level remains high, and I have no nausea or fatigue. I work part of the day in the office and leave at 1 PM to prepare and finish packing for my New York City meeting at our agency's office. I receive a text at 5 PM that my trip to NYC has been canceled. Although I am relieved based on the physical toll this may have taken, I was looking forward to this meeting. I'm bummed, but happy that I don't have to make the drive and take the time away from home and the office.

I began to notice something physical happening during my horn practice today. I have a sensation of heartburn in the middle of my chest accompanied with some pain in the middle of my back, near where the radiation treatment was targeted. Perhaps this reflects the changes the radiologist said I would experience in the two months following my radiation therapy. It certainly is reminiscent of the same symptoms I experienced during week two of my radiation treatments. I understand that radiation side effects can take months to reveal themselves.

Thursday, January 23

It's been quite cold outside. Our outside temperature barely reached 30°F every day since last Friday, and it was down to the low teens at night into the morning. I'll be happy when it starts to get warmer. All in all, so far, January is turning out to be a good month.

I find a handmade book on my desk when I arrive at the office today. It's a gift from the lung marketing team. For the last few years, the lung marketing team put together a "Festivus Day" to celebrate the holidays. This year's holiday celebration occurred in December while I was having my radiation treatments. In my absence, Rob, a member of the team, created a full-size production Louis 2.0 theme! It is amazing! All attendees were asked to pose for a photo and write a note to me in a blank-page keepsake book. They wanted to allow others to make an entry, hence the delay in getting the book to me. I page through the book and see dozens of Polaroids of people holding a red-and-green "Louis 2.0" sign with handwritten notes. It's a beautiful keepsake book. I am so overwhelmed reading each message that it is very difficult to hold back the tears as I sit at my desk. This is such a thoughtful thing for the Keytruda lung marketing team to have done. December was a challenging month, which makes this heartfelt gift from my colleagues even more wonderful.

Friday, January 24

Today we have a business meeting in Buckingham, Pennsylvania. It is a fifty-minute drive each way. Our meeting goes well and lasts about five hours. It is very uncomfortable sitting in my chair that long. My back hurts. Once I am back in the car with the heated seats, I am much more comfortable.

I practice my horn tonight and yet again experience that feeling of heartburn. My breathing is shallow, and I have challenges controlling my breath. I go from needing one breath to play an octave to having to take two or more breaths. Something is definitely going on.

Saturday, January 25

I wake up feeling better today. I have a lot to do this morning before going to my horn lesson at noon. It's raining cats and dogs as Scott and I make our way via the Schuylkill Expressway into downtown Philly. Water is flying over the median into our lane from cars going in the opposite direction. By the time we made our way home out of Philly, the Penn DOT (Pennsylvania Department of Transportation) had closed off all lanes in the other direction so as to pump out some of the excess water.

My lesson goes well despite my breathing challenges, which Jack agrees must be related to physical changes occurring based on his assessment of how I'm breathing. I'm very relaxed. If I weren't, my breathing issues would be related to my technique versus a physical change I can't control. We work on Mozart Concerto no. 3, first movement.

Sunday, January 26

I sleep in until 8:30 AM, which I haven't done in quite some time. I feel a bit sluggish today. Something is definitely going on with my irradiated back lesion based on my indigestion symptoms and sensation in that area on my back. My ability to take deep breaths and control them is affected. I'm okay with that since the radiologist forewarned me that the lesion would continue to respond to the radiation therapy over the next two months. I hope that my breathing will improve soon. I begin to feel a little better as the day progresses. I change the sheets on the bed, which is never easy to do under normal circumstances on a king-size bed. I prepare for Monday meetings and get caught up on some other household chores.

I practice my horn around 4 PM and notice that there is a slight improvement in my breathing. My feeling of heartburn is practically gone. My ability to take fewer breaths when playing scales is easier. Whatever has been going on physically is, in fact, sorting itself out in a good way. My horn playing continues to reflect what's happening inside my body.

Scott and I begin watching *Chilling Adventures of Sabrina* tonight. Kiernan Shipka, the actress playing Sabrina, does a great job and the cast is wonderful. We're definitely hooked on this show! It's a cross between *Harry Potter* and *Buffy the Vampire Slayer*. We love Sarah Michelle Geller! Scott and I decide to start re-watching the entire *Buffy* series once we're done with *Sabrina*. It's been years since we last watched *Buffy the Vampire Slayer*. We're excited to see what we remember and what we don't.

Monday, January 27

I'm having a good day today, feeling close to 100 percent energy level. My day is packed with meetings. I have two very important meetings, one in the morning and the other at the end of the day.

My interview for the first marketing position goes well. I get back home just before 6 PM and immediately take a nap. I wake up feeling rested. I call my cousin, Merissa. It has been a few months since we last connected. I miss her. I always enjoy our chats during our FaceTime calls.

I take the day off from practicing given the long workday and interviews.

Tuesday, January 28

I've been sleeping well. I no longer wake up at 5 AM to check my phone for the time. I did this pretty regularly when I was on a higher dexamethasone dose. Sleeping in until 8:30 AM on Sunday would never have occurred two weeks ago when I was taking more dexamethasone. I do feel a little fatigued today. I am looking forward to being done with dexamethasone this coming Friday.

It seems as though I hit a low energy level around 2:30 PM each day. The low doesn't last too long. It occurred yesterday, and yet I was able to regain my energy through to my last meeting from 4 PM until 5 PM. I guess you could say I had a bit of a bounce back. I have my third and final interview for the second marketing position today. My energy level continues to go up and down throughout the day as it has. Although I'm tired by the time I'm home, I skip my nap and use the time to practice. I continue working on Mozart's Concerto no. 3. My breathing is again challenging. I continue to wonder if this is a reoccurring side effect from the radiation I had on my spine. Something physical is definitely going on.

Wednesday, January 29

I continue to feel some fatigue but power through my workday as I have before. My breathing is still challenging. I'm beginning to feel frustrated as my mind swirls with ideas as to what's going on. I remind myself to be patient.

Thursday, January 30

My week continues to go well. My energy level continues to be close to 100 percent despite the extra energy I used for my interviews and long workdays. I decide that if I get one of these new marketing positions, it could very well be my last career move. I'm happy with what I'm doing but ready for a change.

Friday, January 31

Today is my last day of dexamethasone. I'm looking forward to being off dexamethasone, though overall I've had a good week. Today, my energy level is good with no fatigue.

Kristen and Michael come by at 6 PM as we have plans for dinner. We have a nice time together at a local restaurant. It's good seeing them. They are pinball machine enthusiasts. Scott and I sold them two of our pinball machines—*Jurassic Park* and *Terminator 2*—that we had when we relocated here back in early 2016. Michael did a great job updating each machine to LED lighting, which uses less energy. This will prevent the machines from running "hot." The LED lights will be more efficient and last longer. Scott and I smile at each other, happy to hear this. The *Jurassic Park* and *Terminator 2* pinball machines have gone to a good home.

FEBRUARY

Saturday, February 1

Scott and I enjoy a nice day catching up on household chores and gathering receipts in preparation for filing our taxes. My energy level is 100 percent, unchanged without dexamethasone. I take the day off practicing so as to spend time with Scott. We continue to enjoy watching more episodes of the *Chilling Adventures of Sabrina* on Netflix.

....

Sunday, February 2

My energy level is low today. Perhaps this has something to do with being off the dexamethasone. My body is on its own now. The longer we're on dexamethasone, the harder it is for our bodies to take over once we stop taking it. I spend most of the day relaxing and chilling out watching do-it-yourself (DIY) episodes on HGTV.

....

Monday, February 3

I have my first CT scan with Penn Medicine this morning. I feel great. I have every reason to believe, based on how I feel, that my CT scan results will be good. Scott and I arrive at the Valley Forge Radiology Center early. They are able to get me in right away without waiting, so we are literally in and out. My scan only takes about fifteen minutes. I receive a call from Dr. Langer's nurse practitioner at 3:20 PM. I am at the office in a meeting and excuse myself to review the message. Dr. Langer has two nurse practitioners. I usually work with Susie, but today Vicki has left a voicemail message for me, letting me know that I have a mild pulmonary embolism (PE)[44] in my right lower lobe. I am shocked! How can this be? I've been on Xarelto for the last six months, and Xarelto is supposed to prevent PEs. I immediately call Vicki back. I leave a message and within minutes receive a call from Stefanie, an oncology nurse. She says the Xarelto failed, and that Vicki is

---

[44.] Pulmonary embolism is a blockage in one of the pulmonary arteries in your lungs. In most cases, pulmonary embolism is caused by blood clots that travel to the lungs from deep veins in the legs or, rarely, from veins in other parts of the body (deep vein thrombosis). *Source: https://www.notimetowait.com/dvt-pe-explained ?cid=sem_1128369&gclsrc=aw.ds&&gclid=CjOKCQiAyoeCBhCTARIsAOfpKx jO48tCSwWpZU9M8pXNqAtJhlErnG9sy7r-CXLyHMF9BG96111ptRIaAhczEALw _wcB*

calling my pharmacy with a prescription for Lovenox. Stefanie reconfirms that my PE is "mild," and is glad we caught it early.

How can any PE be mild? I will begin Lovenox tomorrow since I've already taken my Xarelto pill this morning. Lovenox is an injectable blood thinner. It's injected on alternate sides of your belly button about two inches away. It hurts when you inject yourself. I can literally feel the needle going through the various levels of skin. It's not a pleasant experience, but if this is what it takes to avoid another PE, then I'll deal with it. Dying from a PE, after all that I've been through, is not an option.

Tuesday, February 4

I'm having a good week, but breathing continues to be challenging especially when I'm playing my French horn. Playing scales has turned into a laboring process, which is far from what it should be. My recent breathing issues worry me. Can this have something to do with the novel coronavirus (SARS-CoV-2) known to cause COVID-19? I have an oncology appointment coming up, so I'll be sure to share this with Dr. Langer.

Wednesday, February 5

Scott receives a Facebook text from his sister's ex-husband with news that his sister, Susan, was in a car accident due to a medical condition. She was driving herself to the hospital. It was a single-car accident. She passed away in the ambulance. This is very sad news. Scott's relationship with Susan was challenging. They had a falling-out in 2007 after their mom, Evelyn, passed away from esophageal cancer. I was very fortunate to have two wonderful moms in my lifetime.

Susan was sixty-four years old. She was Scott's oldest sibling. Her lifestyle was chaotic, which certainly doesn't rationalize her passing. Scott immediately calls his brother, Mark, to share the sad news. As it turns out, Susan had recently picked up and left her apartment in Florida and driven to Tennessee to be with her daughter, Laura, and her fifteen-month-old grandchild. Scott and I believe Susan might have instinctively known something was going on with her health and decided she wanted to be with her family on her final days, considering this abrupt action. She was out driving and we believe she had a cardiac event, which prompted her to drive to the hospital. We learn from Mark that Susan had a cardiac condition but chose not to take anything because she was unable to afford the medication. She didn't qualify for Medicare yet because she was under sixty-five years of age. It is so unfortunate that she was in this situation. Not being able to afford the medication she needed may have caused her death. Scott and I are saddened to hear this.

Thursday, February 6

My appointment with Dr. Langer is today. We will review the CT scan results from Monday. There is so much to cover today with Dr. Langer that Scott and I created a list of questions. Doxycycline[45] was prescribed to manage my acne caused by Tagrisso during my last visit with Dr. Langer in January. How long do I continue to take it? When can we schedule my next MRI of the brain and spine? I need to request a travel letter for our Orient Express trip to Venice and Paris in April that states that I'm authorized to use Lovenox so that I have documentation for traveling with needle syringes. Next on my list of questions is to show Dr. Langer my ankles so he can see the swelling on my left calf caused by the deep vein thrombosis.

[45.] Doxycycline is a broad-spectrum tetracycline-class antibiotic used in the treatment of infections caused by bacteria and certain parasites. It is used to treat bacterial pneumonia, acne, chlamydia infections, Lyme disease, cholera, typhus, and syphilis. It is also used to prevent malaria and, in combination with quinine, to treat malaria. Source: *en.wikipedia.org*

My appointment with Dr. Langer goes very well. The nurse practitioner, Susie, comes in first to let me know I had a "marked" improvement in my CT scan. Scott and I are ecstatic to hear this! My primary tumor in my left lower lung has shrunk to about half the size it was in November. Additionally, all of my lymph nodes have shrunk with most returning to normal size—without cancer. My spine looks much better. Although my T10 vertebra has collapsed to about a third of its original size, my spine looks otherwise "normal." One might think I would be experiencing a lot of back pain. So far, I'm happy to say, I'm not.

My blood work looks good. For the first time my alkaline phosphatase, which measures cancer in your bone, is in the normal range at 106. As Dr. Langer reviews my spine imaging, we asked what all the white spots are. Dr. Langer responds: "New bone growth." There are a lot of white spots. We ask what was there before. Dr. Langer looks at me, and I say, "Cancer?" His look confirms I am right. Despite our amazement as to how much cancer was in my bones, Scott and I are thrilled with all of this wonderful news!

Dr. Langer looks at the swelling in my left leg. He says to keep an eye on it, and that we will see how it responds to the Lovenox. He mentions taking a diuretic if the swelling doesn't go down by my next appointment, scheduled for the first week of March. He also shares that he will prescribe prednisone if the mild PE in my right lower lung lobe isn't gone by my next appointment.

....

Friday, February 7

I'm so happy that it's Friday! It's been a long week. I work from home. Although I feel a little tired today, my day is productive. So much is going on in my body, based on the findings of my CT scan this week. Scott and I continue to process the good news on the results of my CT scan. With all that we went through since November it's great knowing that the cancer is once again shrinking.

Saturday, February 8

Scott and I work on our taxes today. Oh, joy. This is not on our Top Ten list of things we like to do on a Saturday! I feel a little tired but accept that this is the weekend and I need to rest while my body gets better. I have a good horn practice today, but I can definitely tell something is going on that's preventing me from keeping and controlling deep breaths. I am trying not to focus too much on this and just do the best I can. I've spent years building my embouchure, so I'm not giving up now. I'll just continue to power through this, with hope that it'll get better. As long as I don't use too much muscle and breathe as best I can, I'll be okay. When things sort themselves out regarding my breathing, I'll be back to playing horn like a pro!

Sunday, February 9

I'm feeling very sluggish and tired. My overall strength has declined to about 80 percent. I avoid reading too much into this considering all that is going on in my body. I'm in no pain or discomfort. It's the weekend, so I will take this time to relax. Scott and I continue to work on our taxes. I have a good nap and practice my horn. It is difficult to support my breathing as well as I did when I recorded the Beethoven Horn Sonata in F Major, op. 17 for YouTube during the holidays. I'm so glad that I recorded that when I did. Despite how I feel physically, we're having a nice weekend. Scott and I enjoy a walk in our neighborhood. His good friend Ray from Miami calls him. They've known each other for over thirty years. Scott puts him on speakerphone as we walk. Ray has been great with being there for Scott, even more so since my diagnosis. He is kind and always checks in to see how I am doing. Ray loves cats. I like his sense of humor. He always makes me feel good. Scott and I enjoy our time talking with him as we walk.

Monday, February 10

Although I continue feeling a bit sluggish, I still go into the office. I'm hanging in there. I attend several meetings and make it through the day feeling okay, though I am concerned about how I'm feeling overall and wonder what's going on. I hope that whatever it is works itself out and that I am continuing to rid my body of cancer.

I have my brain and spine MRIs on Wednesday, March 4, the day before my next appointment with Dr. Langer. I expect another positive MRI of my brain and spine showing stable disease based on the ten-day radiation treatments I had in December to my back.

Scott's brother confirms that the autopsy for their sister, Susan, was completed today. It looks like Susan did have a cardiac event shortly before she died. This most likely caused her single-vehicle accident. Today she was cremated. Her daughter, Laura, took care of the arrangements. Rest in peace, Susan.

Tuesday, February 11

I am feeling a little bit better today. I'm still wondering if how I feel is related to a delayed reaction to the radiation treatment or any of the other medications I've been taking. It's always a process of elimination to associate side effects with specific treatments or medications. I practice my horn, still having issues with breathing, and now I'm experiencing heartburn. This does not make me happy. I think back to the month of December, when I recorded the Beethoven Sonata in F Major, op. 17: I felt great! I would not be able to make that recording based on the way I feel now. You have to take the good days when you can because you never know what's down the road or around the corner. This is true in life whether or not you have cancer.

Wednesday, February 12

I wake up feeling tired. I believe my pulmonary embolism is either getting better or something else is going on. Overall, I'm comfortable and feel good. Time will tell. I remind myself that there's a lot going on in my body between the PE and the cancer going away. I am sharing my lung cancer journey at a company medical meeting this afternoon. Although it's an honor to be invited, I always feel a bit anxious as it's still surreal and a strange coincidence to have seventeen years of oncology experience, primarily focused in lung cancer, and to be a patient sharing my stage 4 lung cancer journey. I always get teary-eyed when I tell my story, especially that day when my doctor said the pain in my spine wasn't a herniated disc, but a lesion on my spine.

Today's group consists of medical specialists. They know lung cancer. It's a smaller group, which is less overwhelming, and I share more personal thoughts with this group than I have with larger groups. The talk goes well. Everyone is highly engaged and asks good questions. My dear friend Melissa is in the audience. It is good having a friend there. Melissa and her husband, JC, have been extremely supportive throughout my lung cancer journey.

Thursday, February 13

I believe that what I'm experiencing are side effects from the radiation to my spine. I'm definitely experiencing shortness of breath and tiredness despite plenty of sleep. I feel like I just ran really fast for about one minute. I'll reach out to Dr. Langer if it gets worse.

Friday, February 14

Happy Valentine's Day! I'm working from home today. Scott and I are enjoying a nice day. Although we're both working, it's nice to be together during our workday. I've been going into the office practically every day. Fortunately, we give each other different Valentine's Day cards, unlike the Christmas cards that were exactly the same. It was bound to happen sooner or later after all these years!

I decide to write a letter to cancer. My friend Lisa said she's heard that other cancer patients do this. I think it will be good to do. Here goes!

Dear Cancer,

Never in my life would I, or anyone who knows me, expect to learn that I have stage 4 lung cancer at age fifty-nine. I live life to its fullest. I've always been grateful for each day and take nothing for granted ever since my mom passed away in 1988 when I was twenty-eight years old. Scott and I exercised every day up until you arrived. We've traveled the world since we've been together for over twenty-six years. Each trip we've taken has been as though it were our last. Nothing has changed. Your presence has changed nothing. You failed. All of my positive energy is focused on getting better, and guess what: it's working. I am ever so close to being cancer-free. You picked the wrong person to mess with! I control my destiny, not you. You have no right to invade my body, my life. I steer my own ship. You are on the ropes now; your time is up! Everyone who sees me says "you don't look like you have lung cancer." Everyone who talks to me on the phone says "you don't sound like you have lung cancer." Well, that's just it, cancer, you're not part of my life. You're not who I am. You're being eliminated each and every day. I am Louis 2.0. Louis 2.0 was born at my Curtis Summerfest 2019 recital when I performed Beethoven's Sextet in E-flat Major, op. 81b with my horn teacher, Jack, five days after finding out about you. You're nothing more than a temporary speed bump. You had the audacity to invade my body. You don't belong here. GET OUT!!! Your days with me are numbered. I will soon be cancer-free, and you will know what it's like to no longer exist. I look forward to that day and to sharing with others that stage 4 lung cancer is no longer a death sentence. I will spread the word and share how I got rid of you, how you were eliminated. I will share my hope and my positive attitude with everyone. I have the best de facto family complete with amazing friends. I've acquired an incredible world-renowned thoracic oncologist, medical team, the best immunology biologic treatment and, most of all, I have the most AMAZING husband. I recently recorded myself playing the Beethoven Sonata in F Major, op. 17 for Horn and Piano and posted it to YouTube. It is my proudest achievement. It took stage 4 lung cancer to elevate my musical abilities. So you see, cancer, you are insignificant. You're done here. It's time to leave. You no longer have any rent-free space in my body, mind or soul. Nothing you do will ever defeat me. I will die someday, but it won't be because of you. Love and hope conquer all.

Goodbye!

Louis 2.0

Saturday, February 15

I have a horn lesson with Jack in downtown Philly at Curtis Institute today at noon. My lesson goes well, better than last time. Jack and I work on the Mozart Concerto no. 3. We also read through the first movement of the Beethoven Sextet for two horns, op. 81b. I always enjoy playing alongside Jack.

Scott and I continue to gather our documentation for our taxes. Not fun, but we're making some headway. We're enjoying the weekend. Monday is a company holiday. I love three-day weekends!

Sunday, February 16

Scott and I continue to enjoy our weekend. It's warmer outside than usual for this time of year, in the mid-40s. We continue with the arduous task of completing our taxes. Thank goodness we finish that by early afternoon. We upload our documentation and reach out to our accountant Candy, to let her know and schedule our tax appointment. Now we can enjoy the rest of our long weekend!

I feel about the same as yesterday. I'm tired of feeling sluggish. This is so opposite of how I felt in January. I'm frustrated but determined to come up with solutions to feeling better. I continue to guess as to why I'm tired, even after getting eight hours of sleep at night. Is it tiredness due to side effects from doxycycline? This always seems like a crapshoot, trading off one drug's side effects for another when you're trying to feel better. I'm seriously considering discontinuing doxycycline. I'll deal with the acne. That's the least of my worries. I'll see how I feel tomorrow and make the decision then. My horn playing continues to be challenging.

Monday, February 17

I look up the side effects of doxycycline and realize they are similar to Tagrisso and Xgeva regarding shortness of breath and nausea. You can imagine the effects of taking all three together. Unlike with just Xgeva and Tagrisso, with doxycycline I feel like I have heartburn all the time. The package insert for doxycycline says to avoid taking iron and/or heartburn medication within two hours. I've been taking my iron supplement every morning with doxycycline. My evening dose of doxycycline is taken with Tums. I should not be doing this. I believe this may be the reason I feel sluggish and have had GI discomfort. Because of this, I take only one dose of 100 mg doxycycline today. I do not take the evening dose, and because of this I actually feel better. I did not experience any sensation of heartburn today. I believe doxycycline could be the culprit for the heartburn if nothing else. Experiencing shortness of breath along with heartburn has made playing my horn very challenging. My time playing the horn has always been a very positive experience since I started my cancer journey. To have reached such a high level of playing during the holidays and now to be at this point is disheartening. Hey, I get it. I need to take Tagrisso and Xgeva. I believe that Tagrisso is saving my life and Xgeva is making my bones stronger, but if taking doxycycline is causing side effects that prevent me from enjoying my horn practice sessions, then I'll do without that drug and deal with the acne. Enough is enough. No more doxycycline.

Tuesday, February 18

It's been twenty-four hours since I discontinued doxycycline. I feel less sluggish and tired with less dry mouth when I wake up. I experience a noticeable change during my horn practicing session. I don't need to drink water as often during my practice. Overall, I have more control over my breathing. I am able to support my phrasing better by taking fewer breaths to play a passage.

I am now convinced the 100 mg of doxycycline twice a day since I started taking it mid-December has had something to do with my shortness of breath and heartburn problems. I can always resume doxycycline if and when the acne gets bad. Until then, I can do without the side effects it's been causing.

Wednesday, February 19

I'm working from home today since I have only a few conference calls. With everything that's going on with my body, I should take it easy when my work schedule allows. I shouldn't overdo it.

I'm powering through a potential PE in my right lower lung, a DVT in my left leg, plus the cancer in my body is being destroyed by Tagrisso, not to mention the new bone growth I'm experiencing from Xgeva. I continue to feel better since discontinuing the doxycycline. I take a break tonight from practicing to give my body a chance to rest.

Thursday, February 20

Unfortunately, I was not offered the first marketing position I interviewed for. It's been almost a month and still no word on the second marketing position. Am I to consider that no news is good news? I do know one thing. If I do not receive this position, I will not be applying for anything else. Both of my marketing interviews went well. With all that's going on with my health, I did better than I thought I would. I carefully listened to their questions and answered them concisely. I checked in throughout our time together. I am prepared for any decision. I look forward to hearing something soon. I will take this time now to focus on my health. I can evaluate my career options once we return from our Orient Express trip.

I feel a little tired today, but at least I'm not having any heartburn or shortness of breath. I do not miss taking doxycycline. So far, so good—no acne. My "new normal" has landed around 80 percent energy. Since I'm not at 100 percent, I need to start rethinking my ability to maintain my current daily schedule.

Friday, February 21

Although I wake up feeling good at 85 percent energy level, I spent a good portion of the night coughing. Looking at the side effects of Tagrisso, a patient can have new or worsening lung symptoms: wheezing (yes), dry cough (yes), and shortness of breath is back and seems to be worsening. I will deal with these side effects with the hopes that I continue to improve. After all, what's the alternative?

Saturday, February 22

I wake up feeling rested. This is always a good sign of how the day will go. I have my horn lesson with Jack today at noon. Earlier, Jack and I discussed what piece we would play together for Curtis Summerfest 2020. We decided on Brahms's duets. Brahms originally wrote this music for voice. It's hard to find a French horn version of this piece. I wonder if Jack was able to obtain the music so that we can begin to rehearse at today's lesson. I think of texting him but decide not to bother him, though he already mentioned that he received the music from a colleague this week. I have a good warm-up in the morning before Scott and I leave for Philly. We have lunch reservations at Parc directly after my lesson. It's a beautiful day. I already know what I'm ordering: pancakes!

Jack meets me in the Lenfest Hall lobby for my lesson and immediately tells me that he doesn't have the music. His colleague sent him the trombone version of the Brahms piece in bass clef versus the French horn version. He is unsure why he was given the wrong music. Needless to say, I am very disappointed. I am in disbelief that with all the effort spent, we still don't have the right music. Jack suggests I play the first movement of the Beethoven Sonata in F Major, op. 17 as we discussed. Although I appreciate his endorsement, I explain to him, based on how I'm feeling that I won't be able to perform the Beethoven Sonata. The Brahms duet was our option B. I am so upset about this news of not having any music yet that I almost walk out of my lesson. I feel overwhelmed but remain calm, as Jack apologizes several times. I share with him that I would be lying if I said I wasn't disappointed. After we blast through the powerful opening to the first movement of Tchaikovsky's 4th Symphony[46]—and I mean blast—to get rid of my frustration, we immediately talk about other options. Jack mentions the first movement of the Bee- thoven Sextet for two horns that we read last week. As I've mentioned, we performed the first and second movements of Beethoven's Sextet at Curtis Summerfest this past May. We agree the first movement would be another good option for Curtis

---

[46.] *Music:* Tchaikovsky Symphony no. 4 in F Minor, op. 36. Hugo Wolf and the New England Conservatory Philharmonia. Recorded live October 1, 2014 in NEC's Jordan Hall, Boston. (YouTube video, 44:33). Posted by Ronald van den Berg, February 25, 2015; accessed February 2021. *https://www.youtube.com/watch?v=WsPAXd7VDq8*

Summerfest 2020. I will practice this piece in preparation for my next lesson on March 14.

....

Sunday, February 23

Today is a good day. We have no plans—yay! Scott and I spend the early afternoon running errands. We buy some freshly bloomed hyacinth and tulips. They will add some color and spring scents to our home. We enjoy a hamburger with onion rings at a local burger restaurant for lunch. It's been a while since we've had them. They are delicious!

....

Monday, February 24

I'm feeling fatigued today and continue to be concerned this might be my new normal. Given the battle that's occurring inside my body with the EGFR drug Tagrisso working as well as it has, I'm hoping this is why I feel the way I do. Scott and I discuss this and agree not to make any work-related decisions until after our Orient Express trip.

The stock market is down almost 1,000 points today because of the novel coronavirus hitting Italy. What is happening in the world! This is not good news for anyone. Hopefully our trip won't be affected, and the Italians will have this all sorted out by April 18 when we leave for our trip.

....

Tuesday, February 25

Today is our good friend Dean's birthday! We had such a wonderful visit with them in Zug, Switzerland, this past summer. I wish they lived closer. Perhaps they'll be moving back to the States. Scott and I sure do miss them.

Today I wake up having around an 85 percent energy level. My top three symptoms are tiredness, shortness of breath and nausea. I wonder what these side effects are related to. It's been about two weeks since I stopped taking doxycycline. If it is drug related, there's nothing more I can do because I won't stop taking drugs that are saving my life. I'll just continue to power through as best I can.

I find out that I didn't receive the second marketing position. I'm disappointed. I wonder what my career might look like moving forward. With everything going on with my health, perhaps this is a sign that I should assess my professional and personal goals and make some decisions.

I practiced my horn last night. I continue to adapt to this new "normal." My horn sound is strong despite the symptoms I am experiencing. I'm controlling my breathing better, but I'm still not able to sustain long passages. Oh, well, I'll do my best and continue to adapt to the changes in my body as best I can. My enjoyment of playing my French horn far surpasses any barriers that occur due to symptoms or side effects. Good luck with that, cancer!

I just found out that today is also Jen Montone's birthday! Jen had an interview with Sarah Willis, the spokesperson for Horn Hangouts, a social media venue for French horn players, supported by Gebr. Alexander, the French horn maker. Sarah interviewed Jen last February at Curtis Institute of Music. My author photo for this book was taken in our hotel room at the Ritz Carlton, just down the street from Curtis. Scott and I were listening to the interview when he took the photo of me holding my French horn. The Horn Hangout interview with Jen was live-streaming on Facebook.

Wednesday, February 26

Since yesterday, I received a heart emoji from Sarah Willis on my Happy Birthday note to Jen Montone. Jen replied to all, thanking us, and mentioned that Sarah also has a birthday in February!

I feel a little better today. My energy level is about 85 percent. I don't feel as tired throughout the day, and I'm not as dizzy when I get up. Each day is different, but I'm averaging 75 to 85 percent energy level. I continue to experience tiredness, lightheadedness, shortness of breath and now my coughing has progressed.

My horn playing shows some improvement tonight. I'm able to take fewer breaths and play full phrases. My horn sound is even stronger today. I don't know how I'm doing this, but it makes me happy not to let cancer defeat me.

I reflect on not getting either of the marketing positions I interviewed for. Everything happens for a reason. Now I can make any career choices with a clear conscience, free of any "what ifs."

Thursday, February 27

I go into the office today for some meetings. Generally, I feel okay, but a little lightheaded, and my energy level is about 80 percent. My first morning meeting goes well. I wonder, as I'm sitting there, how much longer I can continue to work. I'm struggling each day to get to the next. I should be focusing 100 percent on my health.

Friday, February 28

Something very interesting happened last night. I finished practicing at 7:30 PM. Scott went to a Toastmasters' meeting. I remember saying to myself that I needed to take my Tagrisso. I usually take it between 6:30 PM and 7:30 PM, so it was time. The problem was I got distracted and by the time I realized, I wasn't sure if I had taken my pill. This is a horrible feeling. Tagrisso is saving my life, so the last thing I want to do is forget to take it. I struggled to remember. Finally, at 8:30 PM I realized that I didn't take my dose. Scott set up an Outlook pop-up reminder on my phone so that I won't forget again.

I slept well last night, though I fell asleep after coughing for about thirty minutes. Poor Scott, I hated keeping him awake. He never complains though, never. This morning, Scott told me that I didn't have any more coughing episodes the rest of the night. I woke up feeling good. I have more energy and have no back discomfort in the region of my right lower lung lobe. I've had this feeling of discomfort since the "mild" pulmonary embolism appeared on my February 4 CT scan at Penn Medicine. Perhaps, now that I'm not feeling anything, it's gone? I also feel less shortness of breath, and I can breathe deeper without coughing. These are all good signs.

We travel to Los Angeles today for an international pathologist conference Merck is supporting. We will have biomarker assets that I, along with my coworker Mike T and our agency, created for our interactive digital booth display.

Scott comes with me for support as I continue to experience shortness of breath, tiredness and coughing. He and I first met in L.A. in the early 1990s, when we were both "puppies." We lived here for our first ten years together and are very happy to be back! We are planning to spend our Saturday doing a memory lane tour.

We arrive in L.A. at 9:30 PM. I don't know what I was thinking leaving Philadelphia so late. By the time we get our rental car, check in and go to bed, it is almost midnight, or 3 AM on the East Coast. I am exhausted, though it is great to be back in L.A.

....

Saturday, February 29

Our memory lane tour is awesome! We've been talking about doing this for years. I'm so glad we are doing it now! Scott and I met through a mutual friend at a gay club in North Hollywood—yesterday's version of today's Tinder! We start our tour at that same club. I remember it as if it were yesterday. I can see the light shining down on Scott's eyes that night as we flirted with each other. That was the first time I saw "that look" in his eyes. I'll never forget it.

That day was also my mom's birthday: November 20, 1993. I know you never want to play your cards too soon when you feel a connection with another person, especially when you first meet. But, as we exchanged glances and our eyes connected that night, my deep feelings for this special man hit me like a bolt of lightning.

§

My dear mom would have been fifty-five years old on the day Scott and I met. I reflect back on the talk she and I had while walking up the hill from the ACME and remember her words that she didn't want me growing old alone. If there is one single memory that conveys who my mom was, what we shared that day would be it. A mother's wish for her son. There I was five years later. Mom's words were with me as I looked into Scott's eyes; he has the same beautiful hazel eyes my mom had, happy, loving eyes. Feeling this way, meeting Scott that day was my mom's wish coming true, her gift to me on her birthday.

After our visit to the place we met, we went to the apartment in North Hollywood where Scott lived at the time. This is the apartment Scott and I were in during the 1994 Northridge earthquake. The early dawn quake measured 6.7 on the Richter scale. Scott's apartment was on Colfax Avenue, about a mile away from the epicenter in North Hollywood. We had just returned from a trip to Miami and Orlando to see Scott's family and friends. We had a great time. Upon our return, the night before the quake, I got crazy in my head. I did the classic pushing him away routine because everything was going so well. You know, push him away before he pushes me away. Stupid stuff. I actually left his apartment abruptly that night. We had planned that I would stay with him, but I needed to make a point. On my drive back home to Orange County, I thought about what I did. It was stupid. I was stupid. Realizing this, I turned around and drove back to Scott's and immediately apologized when he opened the door. That morning, at 4:31 AM, the earthquake hit. I am so glad I went back.

I can only imagine how awful I would have felt if I hadn't. Being with Scott during the earthquake was a defining moment for me. It was then I knew that I would be with him for the rest of my life. My life as I knew it would be different. Something inside of me told me that day we would have a wonderful life together. I deserved to be loved. I deserved to be happy. I finally met someone who truly loved me. And here we are, almost twenty-seven years later! See, dreams really do come true!

The day of the Northridge earthquake, Scott was scheduled to move to a new apartment. The bad news, other than the earthquake, was that we had less to move. His TV and bookstand had fallen forward. Most of his belongings were destroyed. We had his friend from across the hall, Tony, kick in his front door because we couldn't open it from the inside due to damage from the earthquake. Water was leaking from the pipes under the toilet. The apartment was uninhabitable. It remained this way for almost two years after the earthquake.

Our next stop was the apartment Scott moved into the day of the earthquake, located in North Hollywood, on Hartsook Street where it intersects with Lankershim Blvd. It took us a while to find it as Hartsook starts and stops in several places throughout North Hollywood. The Hartsook apartment looked better than we remembered. The area was seedy when Scott moved there in January 1994. The same building had been updated and painted. The neighborhood was better. We recalled the days when I would bring Tiffany, my beautiful Dalmatian, with me to Scott's apartment. Tiffany loved coming with me. Scott let her sleep on his bed. She loved that. She never got to do that at my condo in Orange County. One time, when we returned from running some errands on a Sunday morning, Tiffany was rolled up in the middle of the bed all snuggly. She lifted her head up. She had a wrinkle on her face, you know, the one you get from sleeping on the side of your face. Dogs get them, too! She had been sleeping hard so that when she lifted her head, she looked dazed as though she was doing something wrong by sleeping on the bed. She looked so adorable! I gave her lots of kisses. She was the best dog ever. I really miss her. I remember taking her for walks in the Hartsook neighborhood. We remembered a Ralphs supermarket being at the end of the street. Ralphs is still there!

After our Hartsook tour, we talked about going to Orange County where we lived. Why not, it was only 2 PM, and we had the whole day ahead of us. So, we worked our way through L.A. traffic to make our way down to Laguna Beach. Ah, Laguna Beach, how beautiful it is there! Our Aliso Viejo home was just three miles from Laguna. It took us two hours to get there, but seeing all that has changed along Interstate 5 made our trip more of an adventure down memory lane. At one point we looked at each other and said: What the hell were we thinking? We should never have left Southern California to move to Dayton, Ohio. We quickly knew that if we hadn't moved to Dayton, where I started my career in oncology as a sales rep, I wouldn't have the oncology experience and knowledge I have today.

We ended our journey at the shores of the Pacific Ocean at downtown Laguna Beach. It was as if we never left, though we aren't the "puppies" we once were back in those days. Being there made us feel grateful for all that we've experienced together. We made our way to the Royal Hawaiian restaurant, our go-to place to eat in Laguna back in the late 1990s and early 2000s up until we left in 2003. The owner has since passed away. The place had been vacant for a while until someone bought and modernized it. It was kind of Hawaiian kitschy when we used to go there, but that was part of the allure. We enjoyed a nice meal and one cocktail to celebrate the special occasion. I'm so grateful for the many happy memories Scott and I had here!

It has been at least eight years since we last visited Southern California. Our last trip was during the holidays in 2014. We spent our time in L.A. and Orange County before driving up the coast via Santa Barbara and Monterey to Napa Valley. Today, as we drove north on the 110 Freeway from LAX to the Hotel Indigo in downtown L.A., we were in awe as we looked at the downtown L.A. skyline. I made a comment to Scott that downtown looked like a city in the future with the addition of more skyscrapers outlined with LED lighting. We lost count of how many new skyscrapers were added to the skyline since we last visited downtown LA. A very noticeable transformation had taken place over the past ten years. We marveled at how futuristic it looks. Good for you, L.A.!

MARCH

Sunday, March 1

Today I will be at the L.A. Convention Center to support the digital marketing tools we created for the 2020 U.S. and Canadian Academy of Pathology (USCAP) convention, the largest international pathologist conference held yearly. I'm glad I spent most of the day in the car yesterday, because I'll be making up for it today. It's a struggle walking. I feel like I'm in slow motion. I've never experienced anything like this before. I am struggling to breathe, and I get tired fast. Our hotel is about three quarters of a mile away from the convention center. I end up going back and forth several times for various check-ins with the booth setup teams. The exhibit booth looks great! It's the best since I started my current biomarker position over two years ago. I realize this may be my last conference. I am proud of my work and all that I've been able to accomplish over the past five years.

I am so glad Scott is with me on this trip. I am happy that he and I were able to take this trip together and visit all of our special places, though it turns out that I am more exhausted than I thought I'd be. Traveling is not easy, especially to California with the long flight and three-hour time change. Tomorrow is my one and only day at the convention. I'm already exhausted and looking forward to returning home on Tuesday.

....

Monday, March 2

It's a busy day at the 2020 USCAP convention. Apparently, there are no worries about COVID-19 among the attendees here, as I'm not seeing anyone wearing a mask. There were only six people wearing masks on the plane. I arrive by 8 AM and meet my coworker, Dan. Scott and I met Dan and his wife, Gladys, for lunch just in early January. I am happy that we're working together at this conference. We spend most of the day in customer meetings with pathologists. Our discussions are insightful and very informative. I'm not able to take a break for lunch until almost 1 PM. I head off to lunch alone, but coincidently, Scott is nearby. He was able to end his workday early due to the time zone change. We meet at a nearby Smashburger that I pass going to and from our hotel and the convention hall. I'm tired and not feeling well. I see the concern for me in his eyes, but he does not tell me. I know it's because he doesn't want to worry or upset me. I'm just happy to see his smile.

It's a beautiful sunny SoCal day! It's about 72°F outside. By 3:30 PM, I hit the wall. Scott texts me, and I excuse myself to meet him and return to the hotel to rest. We take a nap before meeting Dan for dinner. We all have a good time together. I share with him that I may be going out on disability soon. I've gone so long, working over ten months with stage 4 lung cancer. It's become more and more challenging to get through my workday. What am I doing? I don't have to prove anything to anyone, least of all myself. I continue to feel fatigued, regardless of how much sleep I get, along with a dry cough, lightheadedness and nausea. Dan is totally supportive. He says he doesn't know how I've been able to make it this long. He admires my courage, drive and commitment. Certainly, his words echo my thoughts. Upon returning to Philadelphia, Scott and I will be making an important decision about my career.

Tuesday, March 3

It's a long day as we make our way back to Philadelphia. We arrive home at about 9:30 PM. Our nonstop flight from California was uneventful, though not many people were wearing face masks on the return flight to protect one another from COVID-19. Scott and I feel fine. Goodness gracious, It's all I can do to survive lung cancer and now there's this COVID-19. Are you kidding me? The novel coronavirus seems to be more than our country's president has led us to believe. We'll look to see how this plays out.

Wednesday, March 4

Today I have an MRI of my brain and spine scheduled back at the Radnor Penn Medicine Radiation Center. It is a very unpleasant experience—lying in the tube for over an hour listening to awful hammering sounds without a music headset. I'm back to imagining the music of Beethoven again in my head. A new building next door will replace the existing Radnor Penn Medicine Radiology Center opening sometime in June. It looks state of the art. Their MRI machines will have music! I'm looking forward to that. I am not worried about today's test results. I know I am getting better. Aside from the symptoms or side effects I am combating, I feel like I'm getting better.

Thursday, March 5

I have my monthly appointment with Dr. Langer today. Susie, the nurse practitioner, smiles as she shares that my MRIs continue to be "remarkable." It's a word I've rarely heard used in association with lung cancer. There are no active tumors in my brain or on my spine. Scott and I are happy to hear this news.

I share with Susie the symptoms or side effects I've been experiencing. We realize that I've been off the dexamethasone since the last day of January and that I have nothing now to combat the treatment side effects. I am feeling the full force of the Tagrisso, Xgeva and Lovenox. I believe dexamethasone helped me not to feel the full force of the side effects and stopping its usage is the reason I am feeling them now. I share with Susie that I stopped taking the doxycycline since it gave me such bad heartburn. She supports my decision. I smile, thank her and share with her that I will deal with the acne caused by the Tagrisso if it means experiencing less side effects of another drug I can truly do without. Susie returns my smile!

Scott and I do not wait as long this time to see Dr. Langer. Typically, we wait a few hours to see him. Today we arrive at 1 PM and are on our way back home by 4 PM. Our time with Dr. Langer goes well. He supports my decision to go on disability in the near future. He offers to provide, upon my approval, any necessary medical information needed to support the disability process. We believe this decision on my career will give me more energy to deal with managing my disease and side effects. Now I will be able to focus 100 percent on my health.

Friday, March 6

I have my end-of-year performance review today. This has been the best year of my career. All goes well. Afterward, I think about how hard I worked this year, especially since my stage 4 lung cancer diagnosis in May. How much longer can I keep working? It doesn't seem like my cancer will be going away anytime soon, as much as I wish it would. It's been difficult at times, especially considering all the ups and downs I've experienced managing side effects and my lung cancer.

Saturday, March 7

Scott and I enjoy our Saturday. The weather is getting warmer. We talk about my career and what being at home, focusing on my health full-time, might look like. We discuss our options and agree to decide soon.

We meet our dear friends Tom and Mare for dinner at DeAnna's in Lambertville. She is an assistant vice president of marketing at Merck. "Mare" is a nickname I hesitated to use at first as I did not want to offend her. I call her Mare because of how much she looks and reminds me of Mary Tyler Moore. She loves that nickname and pretends to throw her hat up into the air whenever I call her Mare. We have a special bond since we became friends three years ago.

Tom, her husband, is an attorney. Together they have two sons. Both are in college. Tom started his own firm seven years ago, and it has grown to include sixteen attorneys today. Mare and Tom are very talented, very smart and very kind. I am grateful to have them in our lives. I share with them that Scott and I have been discussing me going out on disability. They fully support this decision. Just like my friend and coworker Dan expressed, they wonder how I've been able to work as long as I have with stage 4 lung cancer.

Sunday, March 8

I continue to practice my French horn every day despite the challenge. The shortness of breath is really inhibiting my endurance. My sound is still strong, but it's very hard to control and maintain my breathing during my practice. I'm not giving up. The satisfaction I gain from practicing far exceeds any challenge. I remind myself to power on!

Monday, March 9

I have a morning filled with conference calls. I immediately am thrown into my work week and once again I ask myself what am I doing? I've proven all I've needed to myself. Scott and I talk while he's at the airport waiting for his flight. I share my thoughts with him, and we discuss waiting until next Monday to make a final decision. Shortly after our call as my day gets crazier, I decide this is it. I'm not waiting. I call the company that runs our disability program and register my disability claim.

Tuesday, March 10

I slept okay last night. It's different with Scott away. I didn't want to take the time to make up the bed this morning, so I slept on the chair and ottoman in our master bedroom. Great for naps, not so much for a full night's sleep. I won't be doing that again. I fold the blanket and put the pillows away; it takes three minutes! I sit on the sofa drinking coffee, watching the morning news as I collect my thoughts. I am feeling a little anxious today. Scott and I connect as we start our days. I always like hearing his voice. He's so caring, so compassionate. He worries about me when he's away. I am a very lucky guy.

I manage to get ready and out the door by 8:35 AM. I get to the office and immediately start clearing my desk. It's unbelievable all the clutter you accumulate over the years. I won't miss any of it. It takes less than an hour to empty my desk and drawers. It's somewhat scary how little time it takes to erase the past four and a half years. Ironically, no one around me seems to notice or ask what I am doing.

Okay, I spoke too soon. As I am taking my last box of items to the car, my dear friend Kristen stops me and asks if I am okay and if I am moving my desk. I tell her that I am okay and that I will catch up with her soon. As I walk out to my car, I think about how she's been such a good friend. We've always sat diagonally from each other. Kristen has been at her desk since before I was at mine. We've enjoyed our interactions and great conversations over the years at the office. I will miss that.

Today I will once again share my patient journey with our market research team for Keytruda. They are a very talented group. My dear friends Lisa, Kristen, Saahil and Victoria are part of this team. I have twenty minutes before my presentation. I reflect on my stage 4 lung cancer journey over the past year. I smile as I think about my Merck family and how much they support me. I think about all the high-priority business projects I spearheaded and delivered out the door. I'm proud of what I've accomplished during my time at Merck. Today will be my last day of work, perhaps for now. I am excited about what lies ahead.

....

Wednesday, March 11

I spend a good part of the day gathering medical information for my short-term disability claim. The medical form isn't too bad, though it takes some back and forth with Dr. Langer's administrative assistant to complete the information needed on the form. I'm hoping to have everything by Friday, end of day. I must admit it is exhausting and stressful. I can't imagine going through this regularly.

Scott returns from his business trip to Raleigh, North Carolina. As he's on his way home from the Philadelphia Airport, we receive an email from American Airlines that our tickets to Italy and France—my sixtieth birthday trip celebration—have been canceled. Scott calls me from his car with the news. We are heartbroken. The COVID-19 situation has escalated to a whole new level. What's happening? I'll be reaching out to the Orient Express tomorrow as I'm sure the train from Venice to Paris will not be happening. Italy has closed its borders, and France is looking to do the same. We are in unbelievable times.

I wonder if I will be alive to see life after COVID-19. How long will it be before we can resume our travel plans and take this trip of a lifetime? Could there be no more trips for me? I am happy I have been able to make it this far. I sure hope I'm here for my sixty-first birthday as I imagine it will take at least a year for traveling to return to normal or what the world now calls a "new" normal. Wow, I thought I was the only one to have coined that phrase earlier in my journey.

Thursday, March 12

Scott calls to say he was able to reach an American Airlines agent and confirm that both of our business class tickets will be refunded. This was the first time we paid for business class round-trip tickets. We rarely fly business class, let alone on a trip to Europe. Scott was so thoughtful to do this. He didn't want to create any more stress than necessary with traveling such a long distance. Scott made sure that our tickets were refundable when he purchased them last November. We're happy that American Airlines honored our refund.

I call the Orient Express and speak with Jackie, the agent who made our booking. At first, Jackie quotes their refund policy, which, based on the time between now and April 29, would be no more than 50 percent. We paid a whopping sum for our Orient Express trip from Venice to Paris. Jackie offers to reschedule our trip for another time.

Neither option is practical for us. Aside from not knowing when COVID-19 will pass, we don't know where my health will be by then. It's really been challenging for Scott and me to plan any trips based on the unpredictability of my cancer. Additionally, the Venice-to-Paris segment of the Orient Express is seasonal. It runs from mid-March to mid-October. Although October would work, it is too risky not knowing when travel abroad will resume and where my health will be at that time. I share these concerns with Jackie, who says she will pass them on to her supervisor and get back to us within a few days. She seems to genuinely understand our situation. We greatly appreciate her willingness to try to accommodate our refund.

Friday, March 13

We hear back from Jackie with the Orient Express. The company approves a full refund, including our deposit. We will receive it within the next eight to ten working days. It's a lot of money, but based on my May 2019 diagnosis of stage 4 lung cancer, we weren't sure I'd be here for it. It was intended as a trip of a lifetime that we didn't want to delay.

Saturday, March 14

We spend most of the day cleaning our home. It's unbelievable how dusty everything is. The house looks great by the time we finish. We run some errands to increase our supply of paper towels, toilet paper and water. Scott and I enjoy our day together and wonder how much longer this madness will continue with COVID-19. There's been no leadership in the White House. Go figure. No solutions. Where are the test kits? What happens if you think you've been exposed and have symptoms?

While we are in the car running errands, we have the radio tuned to WRTI Classical, and we hear Beethoven's 5th Symphony. Right away I can tell that it's the Philadelphia Orchestra. As we park, the orchestra is playing the first movement. I ask Scott if we can stay in the car until the movement is over. There we are, in the parking lot of Walgreens listening to Beethoven's 5th. The Philadelphia Orchestra was scheduled to perform a concert that included both Beethoven Symphonies no. 5 and no. 6. Undaunted, the orchestra played to an empty house. I have tears in my eyes listening to Symphony no. 5 in C Minor.[47] I love Beethoven! Similar to Beethoven's Symphony no. 9, Symphony no. 5 reminds me of my journey. The four-note gloom and doom opening articulates the day I found out about my cancer. The self-reflection inspired by the

[47.] Beethoven Symphony no. 5 in C Minor, op. 67 and Beethoven Symphony no. 6 in F Major, op. 68. Yannick Nézet-Séguin and the Philadelphia Orchestra Beethoven-Now Concert Series, March 2020 performance (YouTube video, 1:26:35). Symphony no. 5 begins at minute 10:37. It is proceeded by the opening performance of Habibi's "Jeder Baum spricht." Posted by the Philadelphia Orchestra, March 14, 2020; accessed November 2020. *https://www.youtube.com/watch?v=zKWYX5ohadQ*

second and third movements is much like stepping back from an intense situation to examine one's options. The segue from the third to the fourth movement is surprising. No composer had done this so effectively until this symphony. The soft murmur of sound that is maintained seemingly forever, leading to an intense crescendo exploding into joy! This movement is positive! It is filled with confidence and power. It reinforces hope and promises better days.

We go inside Walgreens, and when we return to the car, Beethoven's 5th is almost finished. It was eerie not to hear applause at the end. Beethoven's 6th begins. Now I listen intently as I follow the horn solos. Jen Montone never fails to deliver great performances.

The segue from the fourth to the fifth movement in Beethoven's Symphony no. 6 seems to connect the end of the storm with the sky opening up and the sun coming out. The way the horn solo takes over from the clarinet solo is spectacular! It invites the sun to spread its glow in the best way possible and lets the listener know confidently that everything will be okay.

Sunday, March 15

Scott and I sleep in this morning and wake up to our shiny, bright house! I am excited to play excerpts from Beethoven's 6th. I include the horn solo that opens Strauss's "Blue Danube" waltz. It is solemn and peaceful, one of my favorites.

I send Jen Montone an email acknowledging the superb performance of Beethoven's 5th and 6th Symphonies under such trying times. Scott and I had plans to attend this performance with Victoria and Steve. COVID-19 is changing everything.

Monday, March 16

The COVID-19 situation is getting worse. The stock market is down dramatically today, possibly the worst in history. Things seems to be out of control. Scott and I are under full lockdown. We are hoping things get better soon. Where are the test kits? Everyone should have access to free test kits so we can determine who has contracted the novel virus and they can seek treatment right away before others are infected.

I am perfectly content to stay home, away from people, completely focused on getting better, writing and playing my French horn. Now I can nap without the pressure of missing a conference call. I'm glad I decided to go out on short-term disability last week. I am perfectly willing to go back to work if I get cancer-free and these side effects go away. Nothing would make me happier than to resume my life cancer-free.

Scott receives our American Airlines refund today in his PayPal account. We are thrilled to have received this. I also receive notification via email that my short-term disability has been approved through April 2. Not sure why it's for such a short duration. This date coincides with my next appointment with Dr. Langer. It looks like I will need the same forms completed again with any new medical information since the initial documents were submitted. I will check with Dr. Langer during my appointment so we can avoid any additional back and forth. It amazes me that this is the process. Unless I'm missing something, and there will be a cure for stage 4 lung cancer by April 2, this seems like undue stress for any patient to go through.

Tuesday, March 17

It's St. Patrick's Day! We don't think there will be much celebrating since so much of the world is on lockdown due to COVID-19. Today is our good friend Eryn's twentieth birthday. She is in her sophomore year of college. We can't imagine it's been easy for her and the rest of her family in Switzerland.

Wednesday, March 18

Everything seems turned upside down. The lack of leadership in the White House around COVID-19 is stunning. Still no testing kits available, and now they're saying the lab tests aren't accurate nor do labs have the capacity to perform more than two hundred tests a day. That number needs to be two hundred thousand a day. Countries are closing their borders: France, Italy and Canada. The private sector is scrambling to make more tests available and to increase lab capacity. The stock market continues to drop. When will this craziness end? Scott and I remain on lockdown.

Thursday, March 19

Tiredness and nausea are kicking my butt. I don't feel like eating. Thank goodness for my wonderful husband. Scott makes sure I eat today. I am able to do a lot of household work, though changing the sheets and making a king-size bed feels like wrestling with an alligator. I am completely exhausted afterward.

I read in the news that it could take up to eighteen months for a vaccine to be approved by the FDA to treat the COVID-19 virus. I can't imagine battling stage 4 lung cancer amidst a pandemic for that long of a period.

Friday, March 20

Australia and New Zealand have joined the list of countries who have closed their borders due to COVID-19. Carnival Cruise Line is offering their cruise ships to be used as hospitals. Japan hasn't conceded the Summer Olympics scheduled for July. I can't imagine sending athletes anywhere during this time.

I feel a little better today. Lots of rest is all I can do, along with taking Tagrisso and Lovenox daily. Scott and I are looking to have a good weekend, despite this COVID-19 craziness. Almost everyone is still on lockdown. We have enough food and supplies for at least two months. Thank goodness it's only the two of us. With my stage 4 lung cancer, our biggest concern is me contracting COVID-19. That could be fatal. Despite the severe lack of leadership in the White House, Scott and I remain hopeful that there will be solutions soon to relieve the madness.

....

Saturday, March 21

We wake up early and decide to get out of the house after several days indoors. Our first stop is our drycleaners. We have dry cleaning that has been there for weeks. We're not surprised to see that the drycleaners are closed through April 4. The governor of Pennsylvania has mandated that all nonessential businesses close. We move on to the nearby Walgreens for our prescriptions. They have bottled water, and we are able to get a few other supplies. We picked up garage shelving Scott had purchased at Home Depot. We stop at Wegmans in Montgomery Mall. I decide to go in and stay far away from everyone. This is easy, since the store is practically empty. It's eerie to see how empty the store is of supplies. The frozen food section is picked over, as are several other areas including the meat section. It is suggestive of an apocalyptic episode from a sci-fi movie.

I continue to feel better. It seems that sometimes I have a metallic taste in my mouth soon after taking Tagrisso. Fortunately, that has subsided and my appetite has increased as a result. Thank goodness. I'm less lightheaded when I stand up. I'm sleeping well: eight to nine hours with a one-hour nap during the day.

I'm hanging in there as best I can with my horn practicing. It continues to be my best barometer for how my lung capacity is doing.

Sunday, March 22

Scott and I sleep in this morning. It's a nice day. The weather outside is due to reach 71°F. We enjoy a long walk in our neighborhood. It's good to get outside. There are no cars on an otherwise busy road leading to our development. We go for a drive and stop at a Giant and Wegmans to get more supplies. I wait in the car. Scott wears a mask and practices social distancing at each stop, staying at least six feet away from other people. It is hard to believe these times are upon us.

My birthday is one month from today. This is so far from how I wanted to spend my sixtieth birthday. I am resigned to accepting that my plans will have to wait for another time. My goal: to survive my lung cancer and not contract COVID-19. I would like at least ten more years so that Scott and I can enjoy happier days. This is my sixtieth birthday wish.

I take a break from practicing today in order to get more rest. We begin watching *Star Trek: Picard* on CBS Access tonight. I don't think we've ever watched as much TV as we have since this whole COVID-19 catastrophe began. *Picard* is pretty good. Patrick Stewart does a great job!

Monday, March 23

The craziness continues with COVID-19. The stock market continues to go down. It's just above 18,000, down from 29,000 just ten days ago. It's absolutely shocking to see how much this virus has affected the world in such a short time. Fatalities in Italy continue to rise significantly. Canada and Australia have decided not to participate in the Summer Olympics. Finally, the International Olympic Committee comments about postponing the Summer Olympics.

After many weeks, I finally have a good practice. I'm returning to where I was. My control and capacity increase noticeably.

I'm happy to experience this. I play the *Star Trek Into Darkness* horn theme along with excerpts from Beethoven's 6th Symphony and Strauss's "Blue Danube." Playing the "Blue Danube" horn solo always reminds me of our trips to Vienna. My practice goes well, a personal glimmer of "good" amidst all the madness going on in the world. Playing my French horn continues to be a bright light on the path of life.

Scott has a FaceTime call with our friends Shawn and Grace in Austin, Texas, while I am practicing. Grace is due with their first baby in less than a month. They don't know the sex yet; they want to be surprised. I think it's going to be a boy. I just have this feeling. They've picked the name Sage Grey if it's a girl and Gideon Fox if it's a boy. It's kind of bittersweet to think of any baby being born during this horrible time. At least one positive thing is happening during this time. I wish there were more.

It's cold out, and it rains all day. We watch Episode 6 of *War of the Worlds*, which seems appropriate at this time, and Season 3, Episode 2 of *Westworld*. *War of the Worlds* is moving very slowly. It needs to spend more time on the aliens and less time building the characters. Despite the slow pace, it keeps our interest, so we continue to watch it. The new season of *Westworld* on HBO is beginning to make more sense. Scott and I like it because it's so futuristic. Ironically, part of it is filmed where our hotel was located in downtown L.A. during our trip earlier this month. It looks like it's going to be a face-off between Delores and Maeve, the two main "host" (android) characters from Seasons 1 and 2.

We hear from our friend Cherie today. She is in Virginia. She flew back to the U.S. from Switzerland to be with Eryn as soon as everything started to get worse from the COVID-19 pandemic. They're staying with Cherie's mom and dad, who live in Virginia. Scott and I are happy they are together, safe and with family.

Tuesday, March 24

The sun is out! The temperature is due to get up to 55°F today. Scott and I are planning on taking a walk later. The metallic taste when I'm eating continues to be almost gone. Luckily, I'm able to enjoy a nice rigatoni with Bolognese sauce for lunch today. It's the best meal I've enjoyed tasting for weeks!

The day goes by as it has for the past two weeks. I don't miss working. I do miss my friends and coworkers. I haven't been up to talking with anyone since my birthday trip was canceled. I really don't want to focus on negative stuff caused by COVID-19. My days are spent writing and practicing my French horn. I enjoy seeing Scott throughout the day, though he is downstairs on conference calls most of his workday. I tease him sometimes just to get a rise out of him. He works so hard all the time. I tell him not to take me too seriously. I reserve the right to stick my tongue out at him anytime! 😛

I practice my horn today. It doesn't go quite as well as it did yesterday. I'm managing my days as best I can. Some days are more challenging than others. The COVID-19 crisis isn't helping. I wish we had some normalcy.

Wednesday, March 25

It's raining and cold outside today. This personifies how I feel and what's going on in the world: gloom and doom! Congress approved a two trillion-dollar relief package to help support Americans and corporations, including the airlines, during these tough times. I'm glad that all eligible citizens will receive relief.

It's still hard to believe and accept that most of the world has shut down due to COVID-19. Everything in the world has changed. It seems like the whole world is experiencing how scary it is to live with shortness of breath as part of a compromised lung and immune system just like I am. How coincidental is that!

Thursday, March 26

I feel better today. It seems there's been at least one day a week when I just don't feel well, having less energy, being more tired and feeling more lightheaded when I stand up. Today I have more energy and I am able to make the bed, do laundry and light housekeeping without having severe shortness of breath. That's the biggest debilitating side effect right now.

Friday, March 27

TGIF! The weeks seem to be longer. Not working has helped eliminate stress, though managing my lung cancer along with the fear of contracting COVID-19 has significantly replaced work-related stress. I hear from a few friends today. Most of my days are quiet, so it always nice to hear from friends.

My horn practice goes well. Scott and I enjoy a walk around our neighborhood. The temperature reaches 60°F. I'm happy to be home with Scott. It's reassuring knowing that he's with me. He works all day into the evening, but I don't care because I know that he'll be there if I need him. What would I have him do? Sit there, hold my hand and stare at me to make sure I'm okay? I don't think so.

Saturday, March 28

It's a rainy weekend. Scott and I make the decision to go out early this morning to get additional food supplies. We're concerned that supplies may dwindle as the COVID-19 social distancing date gets pushed out and there are delays in the food supply distribution process. Our first stop is Henning's market. It is way too busy for a rainy early Saturday morning. In hindsight, we shouldn't have gone in. Apparently, many seniors had the same idea. There are too many people in the store. Henning's doesn't yet have sufficient monitoring in place. Scott and I scramble to find the supplies we need so we can get out of there as soon as possible. It's crazy! At checkout, I empty my cart and have to position it between myself and the next person in line to keep social distancing. They don't seem to appreciate this, but I do not care given my lung cancer, high-risk status.

Our next stop is our Walgreens pharmacy. This is always a safe bet since it is never very busy even during "normal" times. This stop is no exception. Before heading home, we make one last stop to get the necessary ingredients to make my mom's homemade spaghetti and meatball recipe for our Saturday evening dinner this weekend.

Sunday, March 29

The rain continues. My energy level this weekend has shown slight improvement. My coughing and shortness of breath have subsided. I took yesterday off from practicing my horn, so today I practice so as not to miss two consecutive days. Scott has been cleaning and organizing our garage. It looks so much better!

Monday, March 30

"Social distancing"—such a rapidly familiar phrase—has been extended through April 30 in Pennsylvania. So much for the Easter April 11 date our fearless leader in the White House was dictating that social distancing restrictions would be lifted. I anticipate this will extend beyond April 30. Our leaders are projecting COVID-19 deaths to reach upwards of 100,000 people. I predict that this number will go far beyond that figure. Where are the tests kits? The ventilators? Where are the solutions??? Nothing. What's the magic number of COVID-19 deaths going to be before we see some unilateral solutions? What is it going to take? Money by way of checks in the mail? Last time I checked, we need to be alive to spend money or have a need for it. While bodies are piling up in the corner, our president focuses more on his re-election and the stock market than providing solutions to save American lives.

I receive a call from Radnor Penn Medicine Radiology to confirm my CT scan tomorrow morning. I need to drink two large cups of barium prior to my scan. This will require two hours. My appointment is for 9 AM. Their office hours have changed due to limited staffing caused by COVID-19. They ask me to come by today to pick up the barium. I tell the staff member that I am on lockdown and cannot make it. Rebecca, the scheduler, says she will see if they can change my appointment. I ask her please not to do that. I will arrive at 7:30 AM and make sure I drink the barium by 9 AM in time for my scheduled appointment. She's okay with this.

This is all very stressful to manage at any time, let alone during a pandemic. I need this scan to see how Tagrisso is affecting my primary lung tumor. I'm hoping that it's continuing to shrink. My coughing and shortness of breath has improved. It will be interesting to see if these side effects have subsided because my primary tumor has shrunk. I've been anxiously waiting for this scan over the past month and hoping that it wouldn't be canceled or rescheduled due to COVID-19. My fingers are crossed that the appointment occurs as scheduled and all goes well with the CT scan results.

Tuesday, March 31

I didn't sleep well last night. There is so much on my mind as I prepare for my CT scan this morning. Is my cancer going away? Has my primary tumor in the lower left lobe of my lung shrunk? Is the cancer gone from other areas? Then, as I ask myself these questions, the thought of contracting COVID-19 enters and I think about whether this could be the end for me. Beethoven's

9th Symphony keeps playing in my head as it swirls with these thoughts. The Philadelphia Orchestra is performing Beethoven's 1st and 9th Symphonies this weekend at the Kimmel Center. We had purchased tickets with our friends Sampty and Kyle. As mentioned, two weeks ago, due to the pandemic, the Philadelphia Orchestra ended up performing Beethoven Symphony no. 5 in C minor, op. 67 along with Beethoven Symphony no. 6 in F Major, op. 68 as part of their BeethovenNow series to an empty audience.[48] (The YouTube link referenced in the footnote is for this concert.) Unfortunately, their Beethoven-Now concert of Beethoven Symphony no. 1 in C major, op. 21 and Beethoven Symphony no. 9 in D Minor, op. 125,[49] which was scheduled for tomorrow, has also been canceled due to COVID-19. I can't imagine how long it will be until we we see more than a hundred chorus members along with another hundred orchestra musicians together on one stage anytime soon. It breaks my heart to hear this. I let Kyle and Sampty know that our plans to hear Beethoven's 9th will have to wait until another time.

---

48. *Music*: Beethoven Symphony no. 5 in C Minor, op. 67 and Beethoven Symphony no. 6 in F Major, op. 68. Yannick Nézet-Séguin and the Philadelphia Orchestra BeethovenNow Concert Series, March 2020 performance (YouTube video, 1:26:35). Symphony no. 5 begins at minute 10:37. It is proceeded by the opening performance of Habibi's "Jeder Baum spricht." Minute 44:13 marks the beginning of Symphony no. 6 in F Major, op. 68 "Pastoral." Posted by the Philadelphia Orchestra, March 14, 2020; accessed November 2020. *https://www.youtube.com/watch?v=zKWYX5ohadQ*

49. *Music:*
Beethoven, Symphony No. 1 in C Major, op. 21. Sir Georg Solti conducting the Chicago Symphony Orchestra. Posted by Ahmed Barod December 4, 2012; accessed by Louis Cesarini February 2021. *https://www.youtube.com/watch?v=Pj2neof3MIs*

Beethoven: Symphony no. 9 in D Minor, op. 125 "Choral." The Mormon Tabernacle Choir, Eugene Ormandy, and the Philadelphia Orchestra (YouTube video, 1:08:14). Posted by soy ink, August 24, 2017; accessed September 2020. *https://www.youtube.com/watch?v=eb_vUFxgtxM*

I arrive at the Radnor Penn Medicine Radiology Center early; the waiting area is empty. It's very eerie to see this considering how crowded it normally is. Occasionally one other patient shows up, but it's not long before they are called to go back for their scan. Everyone, myself and staff included, are wearing masks. There is one woman who shows up without one, but that's it.

I drink two containers of the barium contrast fluid. This fluid separates the GI imaging from the chest, abdomen and pelvis areas and makes the imaging specific to the affected lung cancer areas. I arrived at 7:30 AM as planned and am supposed to drink one container of barium by 8:15 AM and begin the other at that time. I make the mistake of drinking both by 8:15 AM. I pay the price; it immediately gives me diarrhea. I finally get called back for my CT scan. I haven't had this technician before, though it's hard to recognize anyone with a mask on. The technician injects the IV into my left arm. Ouch, it really hurts! Being stuck with needles is never pleasant.

APRIL

Wednesday, April 1

I'm not in any frame of mind to pull an April Fool's Day joke on anyone today. The person in the White House "leading" us is enough of a joke that continues every day. A few of my friends have reached out to ask how I'm doing. All I can do is respond with a few words or a "heart" emoji. I really appreciate all of their support, but I just do not want to talk to anyone right now. The added stress of potentially contracting COVID-19 while dealing with my lung cancer is unbearable. There's so much negativity in the world. I don't have the bandwidth to rehash any more thoughts on the COVID-19 situation beyond what I've shared. I wish I could be there for my friends to help them, but I can't right now. Knowing this further drains my emotional energy. I hope they understand.

I receive a call letting me know that my appointment with Dr. Langer tomorrow will be via telemedicine. This is understandable given the COVID-19 situation. I'm just happy to know my appointment will happen. I am still scheduled to have blood drawn for blood work along with my Xgeva shot at the Penn Medicine downtown cancer center tomorrow. My appointment with Dr. Langer is scheduled for 1:15 PM, but he typically is at least an hour behind. I'll look to arrive at the Penn Medicine Abramson Cancer Center by noon tomorrow so that I can have my blood work done, receive my Xgeva shot and arrive home in time for my tele-visit with Dr. Langer.

My horn practicing continues to be more and more challenging. My shortness of breath, dry cough and constant feeling of being tired have been a hindrance now for over a month. I continue to power through my practice sessions despite this, trying not to panic or be too hard on myself. It's important for me to maintain my endurance so that when I start feeling better my horn playing will "pop" like it has before.

Thursday, April 2

I am anxious to talk with Dr. Langer and learn the results of Tuesday's CT scan. I have no reason to be worried in that regard. I truly believe Tagrisso and Xgeva together are working well. Aside from my respiratory distress, I feel good. It's hard not to worry that I have COVID-19, since "dry cough" and "shortness of breath" are two side effects of the virus. I continually vacillate between thinking I've been infected with COVID-19 and thinking that how I'm feeling is due to my radiation treatment or the side effects of Tagrisso, Xgeva and Lovenox. All three are powerhouse drugs.

As we make our way to downtown Philadelphia, it is astonishing to see how little traffic there is. It truly seems like there has been an apocalypse. It has never taken less than forty minutes to drive door-to-door for my Penn Medicine appointments.

We decide that Scott will remain in the car and not risk being exposed. We park in the cancer center parking garage. There are practically no other cars. I take the elevator, which is empty, up to the thoracic cancer unit on the second floor. I am greeted by a man in scrubs, medical gloves and a face mask. He takes my temperature—97.9°F—and tells me this is my "pass" to get in. My temperature tends to run low, which is probably a good thing nowadays. Fevers are another prominent symptom for COVID-19.

I am called back for my blood to be drawn in a matter of minutes after I check in. I make my way to the infusion side and wait about an hour before I receive my Xgeva shot. It takes thirty minutes to "mix" and prepare Xgeva, plus they have to wait for my blood work to ensure my calcium levels are normal. Because Xgeva is a bone-density drug for cancer patients, it can decrease the body's calcium levels. I've been taking calcium and vitamin D supplements this past month to prevent this.

I am all done by 1:30 PM. While I was waiting, I received a text from Dr. Langer's administrative assistant, Jackie, that he is running an hour behind. This was expected, as mentioned. With the additional time, Scott and I are able to drive home to wait for my telemedicine appointment. Dr. Langer calls at about 2:20 PM. It is good seeing him, and he immediately asks me how I am doing. I share with him the challenges I'm having with coughing, shortness of breath and tiredness. Dr. Langer pulls up the images of my latest CT scan. He, along with the radiologist and pulmonologist, were unable to determine the size of my primary tumor because my lungs are "clouded" over by schmutz. My left lung looks bad. Scott and I look at each other as we realize that the cause of my breathing struggles looks to be pneumonitis. This accounts for the shortness of breath, dry cough and tiredness I've been feeling over the past two months. Dr. Langer is concerned given the COVID-19 situation along with hearing that I am in discomfort with respiratory distress. Though he believes my symptoms could be pneumonitis caused by the radiation, he immediately orders a COVID-19 test. To cover both scenarios, he prescribes prednisone: five days at 60 mg followed by five days at 50 mg, then five days at 40 mg etcetera, until I'm down to 5 mg per day for five days. This anti-inflammatory will provide relief for my lungs and clear up the schmutz. I share with Dr. Langer that my horn playing has been very challenging. He says I should feel relief within forty-eight to seventy-two hours. I am looking forward to returning back to quality horn practice sessions!

No other signs of metastasis are seen in my CT scan. Nothing in my lymph nodes or bones. All images of bone continue to show "white" on the image, reflecting new bone growth. There is now a lot of white! I'm again struck by how much cancer I had in my bones not that long ago. My brain and spine MRIs from last month were negative for any signs of metastasis, so this is all excellent news! I am officially in stable disease.

I show Dr. Langer my left calf; the swelling from my DVT has reduced. This is the Lovenox working. He is happy to see this.

We are on the call for about twenty minutes. My follow-up appointment is scheduled for early May. Depending on how the COVID-19 crisis continues, moving forward I may have blood work and my Xgeva shot given to me at home via a home health nurse. I'm okay with this. It is very important for me to continue my monthly treatment especially given how well I've been responding.

I am exhausted when we arrive home. My wonderful husband Scott goes to the pharmacy to collect my prednisone prescription. Since it's later in the day, I begin with half a dose, 30 mg, for today only. I will begin the 60 mg for five days dosage starting tomorrow. Scott and I reflect on our conversation with Dr. Langer regarding my respiratory distress. We begin to put the pieces together. Thanks to my journal entries, I am able to determine that symptoms of my respiratory distress began on January 18, just after I finished taking dexamethasone. It seems the dexamethasone was masking the side effects of the radiation. Radiation, depending on the area that's targeted, can cause pneumonitis.

....

Friday, April 3

I spend the afternoon gathering medical information from my recent appointment so I can resubmit updated information for my short-term disability claim. I hear from Susie, Dr. Langer's nurse practitioner, at the end of the day. She calls to give me the information on how to obtain my COVID-19 test as a follow-up to yesterday's appointment with him. We don't believe that I've been exposed to COVID-19, but with all we still don't know about this virus, I need to be tested so we can rule it out. It's almost 5 PM, and they don't test on the weekends, so I will have to call after 8 AM on Monday to schedule an appointment that day.

My horn practice tonight is challenging. It's hard to control my sound. It wavers as I try to play. The airflow I produce is erratic, but I continue to hold onto the thought that it will get better.

....

Saturday, April 4

It's a good day today. I wake up feeling better. I'm hardly coughing, especially when I sleep. It's surprising how fast the prednisone is working. My lungs needed a boost to heal. I'm very happy. Scott and I enjoy our day as we continue to stay home. We spend the day making my mom's homemade spaghetti sauce and meatballs.

I reached out to my good friend Erica via text this morning to see if she and Chris are up for a virtual call today at 5:30 PM. Social distancing has been in effect since early March to help reduce COVID-19 transmission. It seems to be working, but we haven't been able to see any of our friends since we've been on lockdown. We had a FaceTime call with Erica and Chris. It was great seeing them. Their doggy, Duke, even joined us! He is a sweet boy with a beautiful jet-black fur coat. Duke is a Labrador mix. At one point, he jumped up on the sofa to get closer to Erica. It was so adorable! Erica and Chris are getting married on June 19. Their ceremony and reception will be at the Please Touch Museum in downtown Philadelphia. So far, it is still on, pending the lift of the COVID-19 city-wide shutdown. Hopefully this nightmare will be over soon so Erica and Chris can have their wedding.

My horn practicing is beginning to sound better. I can tell the prednisone is working. I am able to take deeper breaths and control the exhale without coughing. My horn playing continues to be the best indicator for how my lungs are functioning. Dr. Langer was right when he said that I would begin feeling better within forty-eight hours of initiating the prednisone.

Sunday, April 5

I bought professional hair trimmers this week so Scott and I could trim our hair. All hair salons in Pennsylvania are closed due to COVID-19 because they are considered "nonessential." Because of this, we're forced to cut our own hair. This is easier said than done. I trimmed Scott's hair last week and did well. I only took a little off so as not to butcher his hair. Unfortunately, he had never used a clipper before. His first attempt with my hair yields that dreaded result of a clipper scalping the back of your head. Yep, that's what happens. It looks like a three-year-old cut my hair!! OMG, thank goodness it's only hair and will grow back. I do my best to fix it while Scott holds the mirror so I can see. It is difficult, so rather than make it worse, I stop and decide to just live with it. The front of my hair looks fine. I won't have to look at the back every day, but Scott will be reminded every time he sees me from behind!

I continue to receive encouraging texts from my dear friend and coworker, Mare. We consistently have kept in touch throughout my journey. So many of us have more free time than we normally have since we've been on lockdown, required to stay home, away from people in order to help prevent the spread of COVID-19. Mare reaches out to me via text today to see how I am doing, so I give her a call. It is so good to hear her voice. She is always very positive and encouraging. Mare is very happy to hear the news on my CT scan. It's great catching up. We talk about our birthdays. Her youngest son's birthday is April 18, and Mare's is just a few days after mine, on April 27.

Monday, April 6

I call Penn Medicine to schedule my COVID-19 test. My appointment is at 1 PM today at the Radnor Penn Medicine Radiology location in King of Prussia. You need a doctor's order, which Susie already wrote, to schedule a COVID-19 testing appointment. My shortness of breath and dry cough are known side effects from my medication. Dr. Langer believes that the radiation I had on my spine in December could also be the cause of my pneumonitis-type symptoms. Since they are also symptoms of the COVID-19 virus, we want to be sure there is no relationship.

Scott drives me to my appointment. We both bring our masks and gloves so as to be extra safe. It's a scene right out of the movie *E.T.* The healthcare providers are in full safety gear: coveralls, face masks and plastic screens across their faces as they ask me questions regarding my symptoms.

The test entails inserting a cotton swab in each nostril. It goes way up into your nasal cavity. It is a very uncomfortable feeling. It puts tears in my eyes and makes me cough. It is reminiscent of a prostate exam: invasive and very uncomfortable. This is an experience I will never forget.

They say I will have the results in eight to ten days and will receive a phone call from my doctor if the test is positive. Honestly, I am not concerned. I do not believe I've been exposed. Even if I were asymptomatic, how would we account for Scott not having any symptoms? Either way, it'll be good to know.

Tuesday, April 7

Today would have been my parents' sixty-second wedding anniversary. My mom would have been eighty-two and my dad eighty-four years old. I'm glad they are not here to endure the fear of contracting the COVID-19 virus. It is a horrible death. Your lungs constrict to the point where you can hardly breathe. Severe patients have to be intubated and put on ventilator machines. No family members are allowed to be with you, since you are infected with the virus. This means that if you die, you die alone. To add further insult to injury, in many cases, your family can't even have a funeral. Your body is most likely frozen until a decent burial can be arranged. This virus is horrible in every way.

Last night, my horn practice went well. It was at least a 50 percent improvement from the day before. Today, my ability to control my breathing and avoid wavering notes shows much improvement. It goes so well that I decide to play along with the first movement of a YouTube recording of Beethoven's Symphony no. 6.[50] It is just like playing along with the orchestra. This really helps to build my endurance. It is fun! Scott comments several times on how well it sounds. I'm glad my lungs are getting better. I am very happy.

Scott feels bad and wants to "fix" the remains of the haircut he gave me. I'm not going to let him anywhere near clippers and my hair for a while!

---

50. *Music:* Beethoven Symphonies nos. 5 & 6. Yannick Nézet-Séguin and the Philadelphia Orchestra BeethovenNow Concert Series, March 2020 performance (YouTube video, 1:26:35). Minute 44:13 marks the beginning of Symphony no. 6 in F Major, op. 68 "Pastoral." Posted by the Philadelphia Orchestra, March 14, 2020; accessed September 2020. *https://www.youtube.com/watch?v=zKWYX5ohadQ*

Wednesday, April 8

I wake up this morning to a message from Penn Medicine. I immediately log in to my account to view it. I am elated to see that I am negative for COVID-19!!! I am so glad to rule this out. Now I can focus on my recovery from the schmutz in my lungs. My goal is to get rid of the "clouds" in my left lung so that when they're gone, the cancer will be gone too!

Tonight, I play the French horn solo from the second movement of Tchaikovsky's Symphony no. 5.[51] This is one of my favorite symphonic horn solos. My playing continues to show improvement. I am so happy that I'm feeling better.

Thursday, April 9

I wake up early this morning in a metaphoric sweat with the thought of needing to find out the details of my short-term disability benefits. It's been over a month since I went on disability, and I need this information to ensure Scott and I can manage our monthly obligations that now include my medical expenses. Actually, I should have received this important information by now. I send my disability contact an email requesting a callback this morning. I receive a response right away, and we arrange to talk around 9 AM. I write down my questions so I won't forget any. Scott and I review them and decide he should be on the call as well to hear the answers to our questions. Our call goes well, though I do get a little short-tempered and frustrated during the conversation. There are some details that are still not clear to me. I've never been on disability before. After I express this, the representative

---

[51.] *Music:* Tchaikovsky Symphony no. 5. Eugene Ormandy and the Philadelphia Orchestra, 1974 (YouTube video, 48:24). Please go to minute 15:40 for the famous French horn solo that is heard at the beginning of the second movement. Remastered and posted by Fafner, August 5, 2016; accessed November 2020. *https://www.youtube.com/watch?v=1_BRAcJmHGA*

walks me through the process, step by step, so that I understand what is happening, when and why. I receive confirmation of my benefits and duration. The service agent says I did a great job providing all the necessary medical information they needed so that my short-term disability claim can be approved for the full six-month duration without me having to provide further medical information between now and September 6, when my short-term disability benefit ends.

....

Friday, April 10

TGIF! Scott and I are so glad it's Friday! We've been on lockdown since Monday, March 9, the day I went on disability. One week later, on March 16, the governor of Pennsylvania initiated the shutdown of all nonessential businesses. This includes all restaurants, hair salons, spas, schools, colleges, sporting events and concerts. Essentially, any and all activities that would have people together in close proximity.

There are over 460,000 COVID-19 cases now in the United States and 16,000 deaths to date. This virus has proven to be the worst event any of us could ever have imagined. With all this, Scott and I continue to embrace the new "normal." We embrace our lockdown experience by creating a To Do list of household chores. I don't think I can remember our home being quite this clean!

I continue to feel better. My playing is stronger, and I have more control over my breathing than I did before. I am playing more like a junior in college versus a junior in high school. Last night I played along with Tchaikovsky's Symphony no. 4 in F Minor, op. 36.[52]

[52.] *Music:* Tchaikovsky Symphony no. 4 in F Minor, op. 36. Eugene Ormandy and the Philadelphia Orchestra (YouTube video, 45:26). Posted by ltapirkanmaa2, February 9, 2017; accessed September 2020. *https://www.youtube.com/watch?v=WsPAXd7VDq8*

It was fun playing along with the YouTube recording. I'm hoping to record more YouTube videos like the horn soundtracks from *Jurassic Park*, *Star Wars*, and *Star Trek*. I'm almost there.

I think back to February, when I was feeling somewhere between 75 and 85 percent any given day. Regardless, I powered through and went to the office most of the time. Honestly, I don't know how I did it. Scott recalls seeing the lack of energy on my face as I left for work in the morning. We know now that my shortness of breath, dry coughing and lack of energy was due to side effects from my medication along with the radiation. The combination most likely caused the pneumonitis-like symptoms in my lungs. All of this is getting better now due to the prednisone. My shortness of breath today is minimal based on how much I exert myself, and coughing is nonexistent. Before I started prednisone, I had shortness of breath from just walking to the bathroom. It felt like I just finished running a 5k! Now I can do most household chores, including making the bed, without breathing challenges. My energy level is between 95 and 100 percent every day now. I no longer hesitate to go up and down the stairs.

I had a dream last night that Scott and I were visiting our friends in Zug, Switzerland. I woke feeling that I had to reach out to Cherie and arrange a FaceTime call. It's been a while since our last call. Cherie and Eryn are still in Virginia with Cherie's parents. I hope they are able to return to Switzerland soon and reunite with Dean, Nathan and Jacob. Cherie tells me that she was thinking about me yesterday and reminded herself to reach out to me. There's no such thing as a coincidence! I fill her in on my health, including being tested for COVID-19. Cherie is amazed to hear that almost all my cancer is gone. We talk about when Scott and I will go back to Italy. I share with her that it really depends on my health and whether a vaccine is developed for COVID-19. Scott and I are so happy that we visited them last summer, in Switzerland. After our call, we talk about how happy we are to have traveled so much through the years. We find our-selves daydreaming and reminiscing about all those trips, espe-cially the ones to Venice and Hawaii. Hopefully, COVID-19 will be behind us soon so Scott and I will be able to travel again. Until then, we'll have our memories and imaginations.

. . . .

Saturday, April 11

Today, I wake up with a great idea! Scott and I bring up our new TUMI luggage from the basement. We officially begin to pack for Italy! We began celebrating my sixtieth birthday last weekend when we made my mom's homemade Italian sauce with meatballs. Today we make our signature sausage, pancetta and saffron rotini pasta dish. For-tunately, we were able to find fresh Roma tomatoes and fresh basil in the grocery store. We have to improvise a bit with packaged sliced prosciutto versus diced. The sliced prosciutto tastes fresh but a bit salty. Scott and I stopped putting salt in our food many years ago when we met. Other than the salt, the recipe turns out really well. We have enough leftovers for Sunday and to freeze for another time.

I have our new bling bling "James Bond" tuxedo shirts out along with the shoes we're going to wear. I want to be as efficient as possible with what we bring so we don't have too much. This isn't easy as we're planning several wardrobe changes on the Orient Express train. First, we'll plan on arriving in nice dress slacks and Zegna sport coats. We have our new flashy Gucci shoes. We'll wear this outfit to lunch.

Since last September, when we started planning my sixtieth birthday trip, I wake up in the middle of the night and look over at the night light shimmering through the curtain sheers across the bedroom, to the left of the fireplace. It always gives me a feeling of peace, hope and tranquility. I imagine having this same feeling in the middle of the night on the Orient Express train as I wake up to the sound of the train chugging up the Swiss Alps en route to Paris. I can see the silhouettes and long shadows of the tall mountains as their snowcaps glisten against the starry sky. It's such a wonderful sight to imagine.

....

Sunday, April 12

It's Easter Sunday! It's hard to believe that we'll be leaving for the timeless city of Venice next week! Scott and I wake up to a warm, sunny day. We spent most of our week cleaning our home and doing some light gardening. There's not much else we can do as the social distancing restrictions remain in full force across the United States.

For the first time since we moved into this new home, three years ago this coming August, we clean and organize the chairs and bar area just outside our lower-level walk-out sliding doors. It was so dusty. I use rocks to level the four-top table. Scott and I fill the planters with soil we bought yesterday at Home Depot. We used to create our own flower arrangements for our large pots and urns around our pool when we lived in Ohio. This will be the first spring we've done so here in Pennsylvania. Although there's no pool here, we're happy to have less upkeep, and we create some colorful pots to give us something nice to look at and enjoy throughout the spring and summer.

Scott and I enjoy a very nice FaceTime call with our dear friends Caro and Dano in Charlotte, North Carolina. It is good seeing them. We're all adapting to the new "normal" as best we can. Cutting our own hair, sourcing toilet paper, face masks and hand sanitizer are some of the topics of our conversation. Who would ever imagine this? What times we are living in. We keep saying it's as close to an apocalypse as any of us have ever seen.

After an afternoon nap, I call my dear friend and coworker Lisa. We have a great time reviewing our COVID-19 adventures and enjoy some much-needed laughter. Lisa always sends the *best* greeting cards. She knows just what to say. Here's what her most recent card says:

Be gentle with yourself (on the front cover).

Inside the card reads: *There's so much going on right now. Just remember there is no right or wrong way to move through it. So, feel however you need to feel, whenever you need to feel it.*

Jake wrote a sweet note: *Dear Louis: I hope that you are doing well . . . I'm sure that this craziness will be all over soon. Sincerely, Jake* (What a wonderful note!)

Lisa added a note of her own: *Hi Louis: Hope you are doing well and staying away from germs! We are trying our best to do the same, so far, so good. I'm thinking about you guys often and hope that you've been able to refocus on better thoughts (like spending so much extra time together)! Anyway, Jake has been willing to take walks with me, so he might be partially enjoying the quality time!! (not!) Wishing you guys a Happy Easter! Hopefully we are at the turning point soon and can get back to socializing in person!*

All of our love, Lisa, Gary and Jake

Talking to Lisa makes me feel so much better. It makes me realize that whether this is my last birthday or not, I'm not going to spend it feeling sorry for myself. I am refocusing on celebrating my sixtieth birthday in the same manner Scott and I celebrate all of our milestone events: filled with love, hope, happiness and living each one as if it were our last.

I practice my horn this afternoon. Although my breathing is getting better, it's still challenging to maneuver through my register. I seem to have more difficulty with my high register. I'm trying to relax and take deep breaths. This usually works, but I'm finding it challenging lately. However, I am able to get through an octave scale without having to interrupt it halfway through to breathe. I will continue to power through my rehearsals as this is the best way to exercise my lungs.

....

Monday, April 13

It's been raining nonstop since Scott and I woke up although it is quite warm, around 63°F. A flash flood warning is issued around noontime. It continues to rain up until 5 PM.

As of today, according to the CDC, there are 24,199 COVID-19 cases in Pennsylvania with 524 deaths; 61,875 cases in New Jersey with 2,351 deaths; and 1,625 cases in Delaware with 35 deaths. I never thought I'd live to see the world as it exists today. It is tragic and very sad. I spend much of the day writing. I always feel inspired and fulfilled when I write. After my diagnosis, I would wonder what not working would be like. I am happy that I'm able to focus on my health now without the stress of work. We cannot count on the world today to provide any positive energy. We have to use our imagination to create our own reality by focusing on controlling the controllables.

Well, guess what? I have a major breakthrough with my horn rehearsal! After two months battling shortness of breath and coughing, this is what I've been waiting for. I knew my playing ability would return. I've been feeling better and better each day since I began the prednisone at the beginning of this month. Tonight, I'm able to get through a full scale without having to take a breath. On my two-octave scales, I only take two breaths. I am able to breathe deeper again and control my exit air much better so that the quality of my horn playing is better and lasts longer. I needed this.

....

Tuesday, April 14

I wake up this morning thinking about which shoes we should bring with us on our trip. Shoes can take up a lot of space and weight, so Scott and I want to be strategic in what we bring and weigh it against what we truly need. I'm thinking no more than three pairs each: a pair of black and brown Gucci loafers, a pair each of black and brown Ferragamo loafers, along with our tuxedo shoes. We'll be wearing dressy or casual dressy. We plan on bring one or two pairs of jeans and/or casual pants. We'll definitely be sure to bring our bathing suits. It'll be too cold to go out into the Adriatic in Venice, but we'll look forward to the Hotel Crillon, Paris. It has an indoor heated pool!

This week, Scott and I continue to celebrate leading up to my sixtieth birthday! We are planning on making our orecchiette pasta dish with squash, broccoli florets, Roma tomatoes, mushrooms, sliced chicken breast, garlic, shallots and a dash of red pepper flakes. Oh, and don't forget the Parmesan Reggiano cheese! It's been a while since we last made this dish. It's one of our favorites!

Scott and I are thrilled to receive news that Grace and Shawn had their first baby today. Gideon Fox was born Monday, April 13, at 10:31 AM weighing in at 8 lbs. 6 oz. If baby pictures are any indication on how we'll look when we get older, this little guy will be one handsome man. They will make great parents.

We bought a portable, freestanding, natural gas pedestal barbeque yesterday online. We were able to get a good price. It'll be fitted with a searing area and rotisserie. There's LED lighting on the controls and an inside light. We're excited since we always enjoyed barbecuing steaks that marinated all day on our grill at our previous home in Ohio. Delta grills are made in Southern California. All California businesses have been shut due to COVID-19 restrictions. It's astonishing how much our everyday lives are affected by this virus. It may be two months or more between the time it takes to manufacture our grill until it ships. I have to pay for it now when I place the order. No problem, at least we're in the queue now so we have better chances of an earlier versus later summer arrival.

I need to plan our driver to the airport. It makes more sense to have a driver take us to and from the airport since we'll be gone for fifteen days. Scott and I always like to arrive early for our international trips, usually four to five hours prior to our flight departure time. We will arrive in Venice from our connecting flight in Rome at about 10 AM. Once we land in Venice, we will be taking a private water taxi from Venice Marco Polo airport to our apartment in Piazza San Marco. Alessandro will most likely meet us at the drop-off entrance to the piazza. His gondolier station is located right there. We can hardly wait to see him, Alessandra, and their son Alvise, along with the rest of our Venetian family!

Scott and I are holding to our commitment to minimizing the items we pack so we can avoid schlepping multiple bags all over Europe. We'll be in Venice for ten days and Paris for five so no need to be unpacking and packing every other day; that's why we chose only two places to visit during our trip. We want to keep it as simple as possible so as not to overburden or overwhelm ourselves. I'll definitely bring along my old Alexander 103 French horn. It'll be nice to practice my horn on the balcony of our apartment overlooking the Piazza San Marco and the city of Venice.

Wednesday, April 15

I turn sixty years old one week from today. I continue to shed my life, as it once was heavily shaped by a career. With each passing day, I leave part of who I was behind. My career, as it was defined, will never be the same. I never imagined this would be how I would end my oncology career. COVID-19 amplifies everything. All of our day-to-day challenges are further emphasized by the pandemic crisis.

My friend James reached out to me last week to see how I was doing. He asked if I had a premonition of the lockdown since I went out on disability the week before the governor of Pennsylvania called for nonessential businesses to close and everyone to stay home. I just laughed. Not really, though getting a heads-up from our friend Alessandro about what was happening in Italy surrounding the pandemic may have factored in. I'm finally beginning to enjoy the extra time. I joined Instagram this past weekend. My Instagram posts are centered around music and the French horn. I'm hoping to connect with other French horn enthusiasts. It'll be a great new way of communicating. In between writing and practicing my French horn, I do household projects. Our home seems to always be clean now. It's never been for this long, ever! My goal each day is to make the day as positive as possible. That's all I can do: control the controllables. An important part of accomplishing this is to limit my exposure to television news channels. There continues to be so much negativity in the world of COVID-19. They say it might be 2022 before there is a vaccine! Our lives will definitely be different for quite some time.

Thursday, April 16

It's hard to believe that we leave for Italy on Saturday. Scott and I are so excited! All the planning, all the preparation and all the anticipation will be realized soon. We are looking forward to our ten days in Venice followed by the train ride of a lifetime to Paris!

I continue to feel great! My energy level has vastly improved. It's as close to 100 percent as it ever has been over the past two months. I was able to change the bedsheets this morning without being winded. My cough is gone, and my shortness of breath is practically nonexistent. I'm able to zip through my horn warm-up, going up and down my scales and arpeggios with accuracy and ease. I am so happy! My endurance is so much better. I'm able to focus on reinforcing good form and technique without struggling to breathe.

Okay, I'm going to use this analogy, don't judge me: I feel like a caterpillar in a cocoon that's becoming a butterfly, shedding my past life as I enter this new one. I am happier now than I can ever remember being since my journey started. I write every day without hesitation. Spring is here! The sun is out more. It gets light earlier in the morning and the days are longer.

Our luggage bags are out, and we've made progress with our packing-yeah! I sent Renato a text this week and confirmed that our San Marco apartment is ready. He is the owner of this apartment and other properties in Venice. He and his family are excited for our visit. The last time we were there was August 2013 for Scott's fiftieth birthday celebration. We spent about ten days during that visit. Venice is our most favorite place in the world! It's hard to fit in all of the favorite things we've enjoyed doing there during our visits throughout the years. We love the fact that there are no cars, just walkways and bridges. Scott and I are pretty good at making our way through the maze of walkways around Venice.

....

Friday, April 17

I have more and more energy each day. I sent Dr. Langer an email yesterday to see when we could schedule my next Xgeva injection and blood work. I've been getting a shot in the arm once a month at the Penn Medicine oncology clinic in downtown Philadelphia. I don't want there to be an interruption in my treatment due to COVID-19 restrictions. Dr. Langer had mentioned during my last appointment about arranging to have someone come to our home to give me my monthly injection. Given the remarkable response I continue to have with Tagrisso and Xgeva, it is very important for me to maintain my current treatment schedule. I believe we have cancer on the ropes, and I do not want to let up on our treatment plan.

I hear back from Dr. Langer this morning. He's so good about getting back to his patients. He generated the orders to have me get my Xgeva shot and get my blood drawn for blood work here at our home prior to my next telemedicine appointment with him in May. I am happy I will be able to continue my treatment schedule and thrilled it will be here at home, reducing the chances of me being exposed to COVID-19.

I reach out to Caro this morning. We are able to catch up via FaceTime. It is wonderful seeing her and Dano on our last Easter Sunday call. FaceTime truly is a great way to socialize, being able to see the person as you're talking to them. This certainly is the future now with all the social distancing restrictions. Caro shows me her two Great Danes, Gustavo and Lucas. Her two "boys" are so big! They are practically baby dinosaurs!

Jack and I also connect this afternoon via FaceTime. Last time he and I saw each other was in February. Jack has great news to share; he has been accepted to the Juilliard School for his master's program in French horn performance! He will be studying with Erik Ralske, principal horn of the Metropolitan Opera. Scott and I are very proud and happy for Jack, and also delighted that he will be staying in the area. His senior recital at Curtis will be rescheduled for this fall. Scott and I will be there.

I give Jack an update on my health. I share with him that I didn't realize how bad I was until I started feeling better. It was truly challenging to breathe. Jack is very happy to hear that I am feeling better. He comments on how strong my voice sounds. His words are music to my ears. We plan for me to continue my lessons with him via Skype as he begins his master's program at Julliard. We talk about next year's Curtis Summerfest. Having so much to look forward to makes me very happy.

In less than twenty-four hours, we leave for Venice! We've laid out our things on our guest bed so that we can choose our "must haves" and avoid the "nice to haves." Our biggest challenge remains deciding on how many wardrobe changes we will have during our Orient Express excursion. Here's where we're at:

All aboard!: sport coats, nice collared shirts and slacks

Cocktail hour: black-tie tuxedos

Formal dinner: white-tie tuxedos

After hours: off the rail with bling-bling open tuxedo shirts sans tie!

I came across a book today while I was dusting, *Unbroken* by Laura Hillenbrand. It's a true story based on the life of Louis "Louie" Zamperini. As a teenager, Louie channeled his defiance into running and discovered that he was gifted. He ran like the wind, so fast that at age nineteen he qualified for the 1936 Olympics in Berlin. Although he didn't win the 5,000-meter race, he is known for his surge of speed at the end. He blasted up from practically last place going into the final lap, finishing eighth. Louie ran his final lap in 56 seconds! Lauri Lehtinen, who placed second that year, won the event four years prior, completing his final lap in 69.2 seconds. I used this same technique when I ran my weekly 5k. Leaving it all out there, surging like a shotgun, is the greatest feeling. I always felt like I was flying!

I think about my life and the life of this other Louis, born more than forty years before me. Our only tangible connection is our name, though on many levels I relate to how I imagine his attitude toward life. As the United States joined World War II, Louie enlisted in the U.S. Army Air Corps, becoming an airman lieutenant. His military journey culminated in a doomed flight when his B-24 crash-landed in Hawaiian waters during a search-and-rescue mission. Louie and another airman survived forty-seven days adrift in a tiny raft only to be captured as Japanese prisoners of war. Louie survived prison camp and after the war magnanimously forgave his captors. In 1998, at nearly eighty-one years old, he ran a leg in the Olympic Torch relay for the Winter Olympics in Nagano, Japan.

I admire Louie for looking adversity in the face and saying "No!" The lesson I take from his story is no matter how gloom and doom life seems, or what the odds are, we must be resilient. In this way, I think any lung cancer patient, certainly myself included, might rightly feel a deep connection to Louie and his story of survival and triumph. It's fair to say a lung cancer patient has a lot in common with the way Louie chose to approach life. Fighting lung cancer is about not giving up even when you feel adrift at sea. It's about continuing to fight even during those times when the cancer seems to knock you back. It's about navigating through life one day at a time, in the best way you can, often with grace and occasionally not—but no less resolved to triumph. These past months have made me more and more determined to craft my own narrative. I, not cancer, define how I live and how I die. Tomorrow Scott and I will *live* together as we look toward my sixtieth birthday celebration and many more tomorrows.

Lisa, Gary and Jake all sent me birthday cards. Fortunately, they arrived before we left. I tear up while reading Lisa's handwritten message:

> *Louis, hoping you have a wonderful birthday. Despite these crazy times, juxtaposed with such an important milestone birthday. I hope that you and Scott are able to focus on celebrating what's most important: your beautiful relationship (and) the awesome friends and de facto family who is surrounding you with love!*

Jake's card is so COOL! It's the Cantina scene from *Star Wars* with Han Solo and the negotiator for the *Millennium Falcon* in front of the band. When you open up the card, it plays the Cantina music. I smile as I open it about a dozen times to hear it play.

Scott and I have a pre-birthday celebration tonight. We open a 1999 Merryvale Napa super red! It is superb! We purchased this bottle on one of our trips to Napa Valley. We think it was back in September 2015, when we went to our last Rubicon event at Francis and Eleanor Coppola's winery in Rutherford, where we first met Caro and Dano. We've cellared this bottle since then. It was well worth the wait! Between the two of us, we almost finish the bottle. After our wine, we decide to shoot some pool. We have a tournament-size pool table in our downstairs rec room that we really enjoy playing, though we haven't played at all since my diagnosis. Tonight, our game is on. Scott admittedly isn't very good. He usually wins when I "scratch" and hit in the eight ball. Not tonight! He wins fair and square. The best out of three. It is one of his best matches! Good for you, Scott! Cheers!

....

Saturday, April 18

It's a big day today! We have a few errands to run prior to leaving for Venice. Scott and I finish packing for our trip. Everything is in place. My French horn is tucked in its case. Our driver, Theo, arrives on time at 1:30 PM. We have plenty of time since our non-stop flight for Rome is scheduled to leave at 6:30 PM. This will allow us to relax, without feeling rushed, prior to leaving. As we leave, standing side by side just outside our front door, we look at each other and smile. Venice, here we come!!!

§

On the flight, business class is full. Scott and I enjoy a glass of champagne as the plane prepares for departure. All feels good as we settle in. We can't wait to see our "Venetian family!"

We connect in Rome for Marco Polo Airport in Venice. All goes well. We are enjoying our journey back to Italy! It won't be long now until we begin my sixtieth birthday celebration. Alessandra is celebrating her birthday today! Scott and I sent a WhatsApp from my cell phone while we were in the American Admirals Club. "*Buon compleanno*" we said to Alessandra. Happy birthday!

We arrive at Marco Polo airport at 2 PM. Having been to Venice many times before, we know the drill. We gather our bags and make our way through customs. We exit on the walkway to the private water taxis. They are pricey, but the personalized service right to your destination, along with the beautiful views, is well worth the price. We are let off at a landing in front of the Gritti Palace Hotel. Our immediate destination is just around the corner, where we meet Stefania, Renato's sister. Stefania assists with the day-to-day managing of the apartments. Renato also owns a charming restaurant, Ristorante da Raffaele. He, along with his wife Paola and of course Stefania, are part of our Venetian family.

Scott and I are happy to see Stefania again as we catch up during our walk to the apartment where we will be staying. It's one that we've stayed in before: a three-bedroom, one bath, with a full kitchen, complete with a washer! The location is just a few steps away from Piazza San Marco. It has everything we need. I really like the mural on the living room wall. It reminds me of a scene from a classic Roman picture book. I'm glad Stefania and Renato selected this apartment for us. It has a nice ambiance. We thank Stephania with a *grande abbraccio*, big hug! We quickly unpack our items that need to be hung up, and we are off to meet Alessandro at his gondolier station. We greet with big hugs and kisses. It's so wonderful seeing him! As with tradition with past arrivals, he whisks us off to a nearby bar and buys us a round of prosecco. We toast to our long-awaited return and cheer with delight at the many celebrations we will be having during our stay!

We arrange to meet Alessandro, Alessandra, Alvise and Angelo, Alessandro's father, along with Anna, Alessandra's mother, for dinner at their home at 5 PM. Scott and I stop at a wine shop to pick up two bottles of Veuve Clicquot champagne—our favorite! Alvise has grown so much! He's thirteen now and almost as tall has his father. Anna and Angelo greet us with a *grande abbraccio!* Dinner is adorned in Venetian tradition, complete with freshly caught fish similar to the sea bass, cod and halibut one would find in the States. There's a specialty called *baccala mantecato*, creamed codfish. Anna made it for dinner when we were last here. It's my favorite, and absolutely delicious! We enjoy a few glasses of champagne and wine toasts throughout the evening while exchanging stories of our adventures since we last saw each other. We love our friends here very much. In their company, Scott and I are "home."

We enjoy Sunday with our traditional walk with Alessandro, meandering among the walkways and bridges throughout Venice. We stop by to see Renato at Ristorante da Raffaele and discuss our plans for my birthday celebration. It is wonderful seeing him as we exchange hugs and kisses. Paola comes by to greet us and we exchange more hugs and kisses with her. Remember, this is Italy. We talk about my birthday and discuss where to have our celebration. Ristorante da Raffaele has an authentic Venetian-style décor adorned with an Italian Renaissance sword and knife collection that Scott and I have always admired. The room has high wooden ceiling beams and is very elegant. Renato and his family have owned this restaurant for many years. Renato does a great job paying homage to his father and family by keeping with the original décor and being the consummate host to his customers and staff. Renato and Paola have always been so very gracious to Scott and me throughout the years. Like the rest of our Venetian family, they are both very loving and kind!

Renato is a dog lover just like Scott and me. We're known to share stories of our beloved animals now and then during our visits. They are all in heaven now, waiting for us at the Rainbow Bridge.

§

Today is Earth Day, April 22, and my birthday!!! I am officially sixty years old. I made it. Up until yesterday, I truly wondered if I would see another birthday. Then I woke up from a nap with the clear thought that there will be more. More birthdays and many more stories to tell.

It's a sunny day in Venice! Scott and I spend the day walking the narrow walkways and crossing the multiple bridges that are Venice! We visit our favorite shops and go into Hotel Danieli, a place near and dear to our hearts. Scott and I reflect on our fiftieth birthday trips that we celebrated at the Hotel Danieli, in a grand suite directly overlooking the Grand Canal. Our good friend Claudio used to be the general manger before retiring in

2012. Claudio upgraded our room for my fiftieth birthday celebration in 2010. Even after he retired in 2013, Claudio reached
out to the new hotel manager and staff on our behalf to ensure
that we had the exact same suite for Scott's fiftieth birthday that
we had for mine! We had an incredible experience at the Hotel
Danieli—both times! As I look back, I am so happy Scott and I
traveled the world like we did, when we did. I am thrilled to have
had the opportunity to travel when we were younger and I was
healthy.

I receive a lot of birthday texts and calls today before Scott and
I begin my incredible sixtieth birthday celebration with Alessandra, Alessandro, Alvise, Anna, Angelo, Paola and Renato, who are
gracious enough to host it at their beautiful apartment. The table
is nearly overflowing with different types of delicious antipasti.
There are all different kinds of prosciutto, such as speck and pancetta. Fresh melon is cut and wrapped in prosciutto. This is our
absolute favorite! Veuve Clicquot champagne is chilling in a bucket
along with several bottles of prosecco. This is an Italian delight fit
for a king! The birthday cake is my favorite: white vanilla icing
with raspberry-custard filling, adorned with rainbow sprinkles.
It is simply beautiful! Andrea Bocelli songs are playing and filling
the high Venetian cathedral-like ceiling of the living room. Outside, the sun is shining and as it sets, we move to the rooftop terrace to enjoy the view.

Everyone is so happy. They comment on how good I look and
are thrilled that I'm winning my fight with cancer. Cancer has
met its match with me, they say.

§

Throughout the day, Scott gives me three birthday cards.
I receive the first one in the morning. It has the number "60"
in front of a wine bottle on the front cover. The inside message
reads: "Wishing you a vintage year. Hope your birthday is rich
and flavorful, accented with a little sparkle, some sassiness, and

a bright finish." Scott writes his own message, and I will share it with you.

> *I already received my wish; "you" are here with me by my side—to feel healthy and safe! Love always, forever yours, Scotty Boo Boo*

This is so adorable of him to write as if it were his birthday. I'll take it. He gives me card number two after our group celebration. There are two Golden Retrievers snuggling on the cover: "For the Man I Love. We have a romance that's sweet, silly, sometimes different and always exactly what we need." Inside is another message from Scott:

> *We know each other, and we trust each other. That's why sharing life with you makes every day mean so much more . . . The journey you've been through says it all. How brave and strong you are. And through it all, you're still standing tall! Love you so many years more like I never have before. Happy 60th birthday!*

> *—With all my love and admiration, Scotty*

I couldn't wish for anything better on this day than being with the love of my life after a day spent celebrating with our friends.

Scott's third card is the *best* ever: "60 Years Amazing, 60 Years Loved."

> *What you've given the world is immeasurable. What you've still got to give is incredible. What we're celebrating about you today is everything wonderful. Hope you spend this birthday enjoying the things that come from living fully and generously, year after amazing year.*

> *Happy birthday! We are with you always.*

> *—Tiffany, Casper, Lance & Amadeus*

It was so precious and very special for Scott to do this. Signing using the names of our beloved pets who are no longer with us is one of many examples, some of which I've already shared, of how amazing Scott is. I truly am one lucky guy! I am extremely grateful for all of my friends on both sides of the Atlantic. Celebrating my sixtieth birthday surrounded by so much love and support means the world to me.

§

Happy day after my birthday! I wake up with the feeling that something has changed inside my body. Am I cancer free? It doesn't matter. I feel great!!! The timing couldn't be better! My energy level is above 100 percent! I have so much energy! I am no longer winded when I go upstairs. I am sleeping well! My appetite is good. I probably could stand to lose a few pounds though!

We spend the rest of the week, into the weekend, continuing our celebration. We enjoy dinners at our favorite restaurants. Renato and Paola's restaurant, Ristorante da Raffaele, is our special favorite. L'Osteria di Santa Marina is another favorite. Our friends Augustino and Caterina co-own L'Osteria di Santa Marina with Danilo and Betty. As with Renato and Paola, they always make us feel welcome, like family whenever we dine there.

We continue to explore the maze of narrow walkways that surround Venice. Oftentimes, everything looks the same, but that's what makes it interesting and fun. There's nothing like crossing a bridge while a gondolier and his gondola go underneath with a family on board. The gondolier is singing, "O Sole Mio" in true Venetian tradition. They're all such good singers, and their voices are always in tune!

On Monday, Scott and I leave for an overnight trip to the Collio wine region. Collio, near the Slovenian border, is about an hour and a half train ride from Venice. Our favorite Italian winery, Schiopetto, is located there. We last visited Maria Angela Schiopetto, along with Carlo and Giorgio, her twin brothers, when we celebrated Scott's fiftieth birthday. Maria Angela and her brothers work hard to produce very fine wines as a tribute to their father, Mario, who passed away in 2003. I recently read that six years ago, in 2014, the Schiopetto winery was passed into the hands of the Rotolo family, who intend to maintain intact Mario's mission and productive philosophy for the sake of continuity.

We look forward to dinner tonight at La Tavernetta. We especially enjoy our dinners there. It's a tavern-like building that houses the restaurant and half a dozen rooms just down the hill from the Roman-era castle on the hill, Castello di Spessa, with its iconic watchtower and majestically landscaped grounds. We've stayed at the tavern before during one of our overnight trips here from Venice. The castle grounds are absolutely gorgeous this time of year. There is a "tunnel" walkway made up of a long arched trellis filled with gorgeous blossoming wisteria. The wisteria is in full bloom; their fragrance is exquisite!

During our last visit to Collio, Scott and I went for 5k run. We used to enjoy a 5k run whenever we traveled. It gave us the opportunity to soak in the wonderful sights. We won't be running during this trip. This was our first time staying at the castle. We always laugh when we relive what happened during that trip. I got lost during my 5k run. All the winding streets of Collio looked the same. All arrows seemed to point to Rome. It was right out of the movies. It was so hot that day I decided to run shirtless. All I had with me was my running shorts and my Apple iPod-Nano with headphones, no cell phone. I ended up heading out of town instead of back to the castle. Once I realized this, I was able to get my bearings and adjust my direction. It took a while, but finally I saw the local golf course, which interweaves with the castle grounds, so I knew it was nearby. As I was heading back, I realized that Scott must have been worried that I hadn't returned yet. This upset me a lot, and I panicked. Already exhausted from an extended run, I kicked in my speed anyway so as to return sooner rather than later. As soon as I reached the castle, a woman in the gift shop greeted me and told me that she had arranged a bicycle for Scott. I was so thrilled to see him when he returned a few minutes later. He thought I had been kidnapped! Needless to say, my 5k run was more of a 10k!

I digress. After a much-needed nap, Scott and I head to dinner at La Tavernetta. They serve Schiopetto wines, so we are able to select some nice food pairings to accompany their exceptional wines. The restaurant is known for their variety of Italian wines, but the Schiopetto red, Podere dei Blumeri, is a wine to be reckoned with. It's a blend of Merlot and Refosco dal Peduncolo Rosso. We choose the 2017 Podere dei Blumeri Schiopetto to go with our dinner.

Our meal begins with an array of tempting appetizers: Saporito delle Valli, a delicious local cheese; pumpkin cream; and artichokes with black truffle slices. The artichokes are in season this time of year, so they are extra delicious! Our main dish is carob fettuccine with dried tomatoes and local sausage. Everything is very yummy! The meal pairs beautifully with our wine choice.

After our nice getaway in Collio, we arrive back in Venice the next afternoon. It's a sunny day today! We are beginning to feel sad knowing that we'll be leaving in a few days, so we make the most of it. We decide to spend our final day here fishing with our dear friend Alessandro. He loves to fish! Squid is in season. Fishing with Alessandro is a tradition we started back in 2010. We enjoy a leisurely lunch at a local restaurant before we head out. I have never tasted artichokes that were so delicious. They actually grow their own. We linger over lunch, complete with prosecco, before heading out to the waterways to fish. Scott and I are a bit tipsy by the time we get there. This makes for a very interesting fishing experience. You have to be careful when you go to remove the squid from your fishing hook. They may spit out black ink, which, as you can imagine, is a stain that will be quite difficult to get out. Luckily, Scott and I are able to avoid any "ink" situation. We've done this before, during my fiftieth birthday trip. It seems that my singing, "here fishy, fishy" works just as well now as it did then because I end up catching the most squid again! At the end of our day together, Scott and I join Alessandra, Alvise and Alessandro for pizza. We have a wonderful time. Although we are sad to be leaving, we enjoy our last day in Venice very much!

§

It's time for our trip of a lifetime train ride aboard the Orient Express! We will be picked up from our Venice apartment at 9:30 AM on Wednesday, April 29. The Orient Express offers door-service pickup and drop-off. This ensures all passengers arrive in time and get safely to their destinations.

We arrive at the train at precisely 10 AM. The train is magnificent! Right out of a 1925 photo book. It's a black train with gold lettering on the top of each car: *Venice-Simplon-Orient Express* (VSOE).[53] Perfectly mannered staff, standing poised in a row across the platform in front of the train, wait to greet us. All are wearing white gloves. This is certain to be a decadent experience. As Scott and I are escorted to our suite, we marvel at the nostalgic décor. We immediately notice the vintage Lalique crystal lamps that line the hallway to the sleeping cars. They are absolutely stunning. No expense has been spared to re-create the nostalgia of this luxury train. Our suite is in the last train car. The three grand suites—"Paris," "Venice" and "Istanbul"—are all located at the end to ensure privacy. We enter the Venice suite and gasp at the furnishings. The décor is gorgeous! The sitting area is nicely separated from the sleeping room. There's plenty of room for us to lounge around and relax. The suite offers a wall of windows that are certain to deliver once-in-a-lifetime views of the Italian-Swiss Alps and French country-side on our way to Paris.

The décor is classic Venetian. All the glass fixtures and appointments are Murano glass. The best representation of this is in the bathroom. The sink is a large cobalt blue Murano bowl. Absolutely beautiful! There's a pan showerhead in the spacious shower, and

---

53. For some highlights about the Venice-Simplon-Orient Express, visit Belmond Management Ltd.: *https://www.belmond.com/trains/europe/venice-simplon-orient -express/* and The Orient Express Grand Suites: *https://www.belmond.com/trains/ europe/venice-simplon-orient-express/grand-suites*

there are plenty of amenities: lotion, soap, bath gel, shampoo and conditioner, a high-end brand with a fragrance of sophistication.

Frederico will be our personal valet during our trip. He is from Verona and has been with VSOE for five years. He is polished and extremely professional with an unpretentious demeanor. He offers to assist us with unpacking, but Scott and I are practically giddy taking all this in. We tip him well before he leaves as we have no problem doing this ourselves. There's plenty of room to unpack our things with ample space to store our luggage.

We relax and enjoy a perfectly chilled glass of champagne as the train prepares to depart Santa Lucia, Venice station for Paris at promptly 11 AM. Taittinger is the champagne of choice for VSOE. We scheduled a late lunch for 3 PM, so we have plenty of time to "chill-lax" as the train gets underway. After enjoying a glass of champagne, we venture out of our room to explore the train. We have a very long walk to the dining area. There are at least a dozen compartment cars that make up this train. Scott and I do not mind the walk. We will be eating plenty and look forward to the exercise. I feel great.

Lunch is chef-prepared with carefully chosen ingredients. Belmond had asked us to share any allergies or dislikes. They are so efficient. Scott and I are in good shape as we excitedly await our first meal. We arrive at our table and are immediately greeted by our server, Michelle, who reviews our menu items. The sommelier stops by and we choose a French Sauternes, one of our favorite white wines, to pair with our meal. Michelle supports our decision and is enthusiastic to hear our choice.

Lunch is wonderfully decadent. The courses are paced out perfectly! There's no rush here on the Orient Express train. The scenery is just as we imagined: breathtakingly gorgeous! The Italian Alps are snowcapped and majestic. The wisteria is in full bloom along with an array of apple, cherry and pear blossoming trees. Sheep are grazing on the hillsides as the sun glistens over fields of lush greenery.

Our meal begins with an Asian fragrance that consists of grilled beef on vegetable salad with Thai dressing. All of the salad ingredients are fresh. You can tell that every item was carefully chosen based on the perfect blend of flavors. Our salad is followed by an aromatic steamed cod and fresh leek salad with egg tofu, shiitake mushroom and spinach. A medley of chocolate and Pandan mousse on crunchy hazelnut praline with orange segment and coconut coulis awaits us for dessert! Yummy! Mignardises (tiny sweets!) are provided as an aperitif (as if we haven't had enough to eat already), which we enjoy with a nice cup of tea with lemon. We venture out from our lunch to enjoy a walk along the train cars. If lunch is this good, we can only imagine what's waiting for us for dinner!

After a long walk back and forth a few times through the train car hallways, we retire to our suite for a nap. I'm not wasting any more time than necessary sleeping on this train experience. We have a long night ahead of us, so a few catnaps should be all we need to be ready to absorb all of our VSOE experience! We wake at 5 PM. We scheduled a late dinner with seating at 9 PM. Scott and I get ready so that we can enjoy a cocktail in the bar before dinner. We don our black-tie tuxedo attire. Now we're ready to enjoy a true "James Bond" experience, aboard the Orient Express Train! Scott and I enjoy our cocktails—"shaken, not stirred" 😆—and are soon on our way to dinner.

Our dinner menu looks amazing! The menu is in French, but I'll provide the English version here. We begin with sea bass fillet roasted with Guerande sea salt, presented on sliced red endives and lentils purée with Venetian clam broth. Next comes spice-braised lamb shank and ewe cheese cream with lemon thyme. A trio of bell peppers with artichoke, Ratte potatoes and spinach filling follows. Durum wheat pasta sprinkled with grated Parmesan cheese and tomatoes completes our main repast before the final courses are served. We select a superb bottle of 2007 Beaucastel Châteauneuf-du-Pape to pair with our dinner. This is especially appreciated with the selection of fine cheeses that arrive! Dessert is especially decadent. Scott and I literally moan as we enjoy the chestnut Mont Blanc, complete with bourbon and vanilla-flavored custard. Mignardises are once again served with freshly ground coffee served in a French press. Scott and I enjoy a few cups of freshly brewed coffee with our dessert. We want to be sure to be awake to enjoy the after-dinner festivities in the bar, complete with live music played on a baby grand. We are glowing from our birthday celebration experience so far!

After dinner, we take another stroll up and down the train car hallways. We enjoy a glass of Taittinger champagne from the unlimited bottles provided as part of our Grand Parlor suite amenities. By this time, we are a bit tipsy. We hydrate to offset the alcoholic effects.

Scott and I return to the bar and continue to be giddy as we live out the events of our Orient Express experience. There is no loss of characters on this train, and I mean that in a very good way because we are among them! We pretend we're in a James Bond movie sipping our martinis, laughing together as we say things you'd expect James Bond to say. At this point I've asked the bartender to water down our drinks, otherwise they'll be peeling us off the floor by the end of our night. We continue to drink lots of water, which helps us maintain a nice buzz versus total intoxication! I can't remember us laughing as hard and as much as we did tonight. We are having the time of our lives!

It's almost 1:30 AM as we make our way back to our suite. It's been an amazing day. We stumble a bit as we undress, continuing to laugh. Scott slips into bed as I make my way to the desk. This is my favorite time of day to write, the early morning hours just before the sun rises. The moonlight reflecting off the beautiful Swiss Alps fills our suite as Scott lies facing me. He sleeps closer and closer to me now. Lately, whenever I wake in the middle of the night, he's right there. I like this. I'm not going anywhere. I feel good. I have no regrets. I've had a rich life. Ever since I met my husband, my Scott, my life has been a beautiful dream come true. All that I have hoped for, all that I ever wanted to do, I've done with this wonderful man. I accept, with a full heart, what lies ahead.

Everything is beautiful and still. Scott wakes up and smiles as I look over at him. There's that look again. I smile back, feeling tears well up as we look intently into each other's eyes. Without saying a word, he knows what just happened. I finished writing the book you are holding in your hands. I am overwhelmed with tears of happiness realizing that I just finished writing my book aboard the Orient Express.

§

I remember the nightlight, next to the fireplace in our bedroom, evoking feelings of peace, hope and tranquility as I begin to doze off. *I awake in our bed at home.* I reach over and hold Scott tight. My heart is full and at peace. I am loved more by this man than I ever dreamed I would be loved by anyone. I won life's grand prize! Scott is the love of my life. He knows this. I reflect on all the love and support I have received from Scott and so many people. They helped me stand up when I stumbled and continue to be a lifeline to this day. I am very grateful. All of the events in my life have led me to this moment. My soul is free, and I'm flying high, conquering life's biggest challenge. I welcome today, knowing this day and every day will be as wonderful as its predecessor. I will live as I've lived before. I couldn't have *imagined* a more wonderful sixtieth birthday celebration![54]

[54.] Beethoven: Symphony no. 9 in D Minor, op. 125 "Choral." The Mormon Tabernacle Choir, Eugene Ormandy and the Philadelphia Orchestra (YouTube video, 1:08:14). Please go to minute 1:06:34 for the dramatic ending of the triumphal 4th movement and remember to "Believe." Posted by soy ink, August 24, 2017; accessed September 2020. *https://www.youtube.com/watch?v=eb_vUFxgtxM*

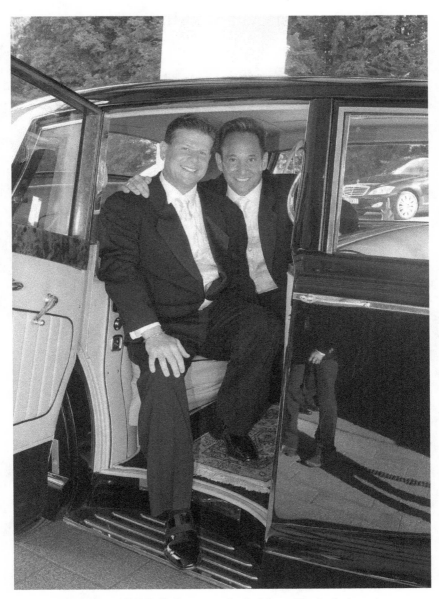

A magical trip in a 1957 Rolls Royce at the Salzburg Festival, Austria, August 2013

MISCELLANEOUS PICTURES

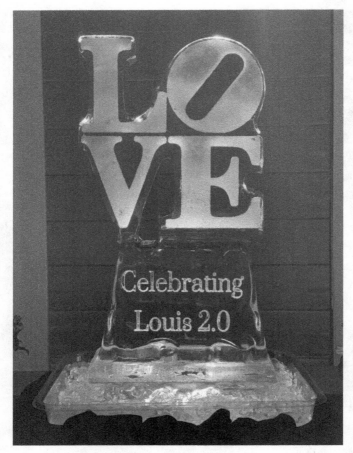

LOVE sign ice sculpture from our Celebration of Life, Love and Friendship event, November 2019

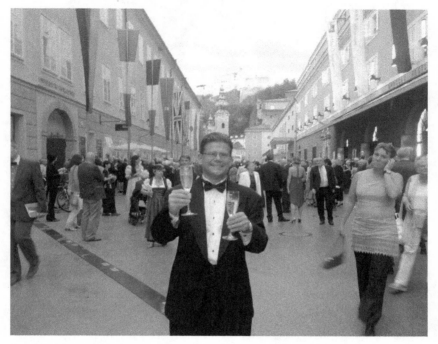

Scott holding champagne glasses at intermission during the Wagner opera Die Meistersinger von Nürnberg on his fiftieth birthday at the Salzburg Festival, Austria, August 2013

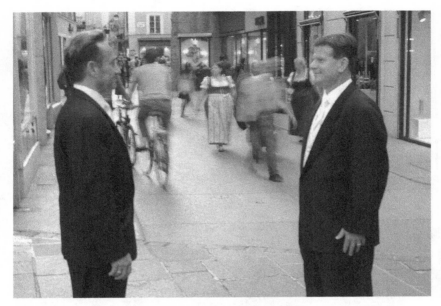

The cobblestone streets of Old Town Salzburg, Austria, August 2013

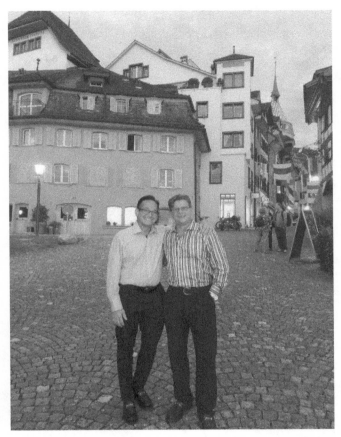

Outside Fischmärt Restaurant in Zug, Switzerland, July 2019

Postscript

I t's been several months since I finished writing *Survival Symphony*. COVID-19 continues to rage through the United States and beyond. Little did Scott and I know last New Year's Eve how tragic 2020 would be. Our country continues to struggle to get COVID-19 under control with over 26 million cases and 451,000 deaths. When will this be over?

March 2020 ended up being the worst month of my life, even compared to when I was diagnosed with stage 4 non-small cell lung cancer in May 2019. I ended up having COVID-19–like symptoms that fortunately were not. I've never been so scared. Scott and Dr. Langer were there every step of the way to maintain my cancer care without interruption. Penn Medicine was on the forefront of patient care so as to ensure ventilators would be available for all COVID-19 patients.

It seems that my use of "new normal" and "believe" became popular with COVID-19. My sixtieth birthday celebration trip became a COVID-19 casualty. Fortunately, I'm doing well considering all of the challenges of having stage 4 lung cancer in a COVID-19 world. I had originally planned on completing this book on the Orient Express train from Venice to Paris. This came to an end with COVID-19. I was heartbroken with all that was happening as the thought that I might not be around for any more trips tore through my heart. COVID-19 changed everything. I rose up and kept with the plan by taking our trip and ending my book virtually. Scott and I have been to Venice many times as we consider it our second home since our first visit in 1997. I've imagined what our experience on the Orient Express would be like through all the planning Scott and I had done. Paris is another one of our favorite places. We're very fortunate to have celebrated several birthdays there as well. There is nothing like celebrating an April birthday in Paris! It was the memory of those previous trips, along with my imagination, that provided the details to virtually create my Sixtieth Birthday Celebration trip.

I hope that you liked my virtual ending. In this day of so much uncertainty with COVID-19, I wanted to share the power of imagination. However many restrictions we have today, nothing, I mean nothing, can stop our imaginations from creating a positive environment or alternate reality to help us cope with living in such challenging times. Hey, it's a day-to-day challenge managing through the ups and downs of today's world. For me, having cancer during these times presented an additional challenge. So, whatever works. This way of thinking helps me a lot.

Remember that pain in my back that I thought was a herniated disc but ended up being a tumor? Well, the good news is that the tumor is gone. The bad news is that two-thirds of my T10 vertebra, where it was located, is also gone. The cancer ate away at the bone, causing my T10 to compress. "Compress" is a fancy word for collapse! I had a vertebroplasty procedure done this summer. For months I had been experiencing back pain, but my scans showed no tumors on my back, so how could this be? When we break bones, we experience a lot of pain. This is no different. My nerve endings were responding to the bone deterioration as if it were a broken bone. I was in a constant 6-out-of-10 on the pain scale, every day. My horn playing further exacerbated the pain. This is where I drew the line! I still rarely take pain medication. My ability to tolerate pain gives me a high pain threshold. Since they don't give out gold medals for how well or how long a person can tolerate pain, I finally made the decision to move forward with the vertebroplasty procedure. Although my recovery lasted about a month, it was the best thing I ever did. No more back pain. Well, maybe about 5 percent. I can breathe better, especially when I play my horn—yeah!

Speaking of my horn playing, in this book I often referred to various practice sessions on a scale of high school or college level. I'm happy to share that I have been consistently playing at the graduate school level of a French Horn Performance major. I am currently working on the Glière Horn Concerto. It's a standard repertoire piece that somehow was left out of my college experience. Learning this beautiful concerto, after so many years, has been very inspiring. The melodies are gorgeous. Perhaps I'll learn a movement or two well enough to record and post on YouTube. Wouldn't that be wonderful.

Scott and I purchased a NordicTrack iFIT bicycle and treadmill this summer. It's been wonderful experiencing long walks around the world virtually, especially in this day of COVID-19. It's very convenient to have this equipment here in our home, at room temperature and safe. I continue to walk two miles a day. I've walked all over the world: in Hawaii, Bora Bora, Costa Rica, the Grand Canyon, Machu Picchu, Slovenia, Italy and Croatia, to name a few. It's such a great virtual experience. A special shout-out to John Peel, iFIT instructor. John is very motivating and extremely positive.

Little did I know that attending the 2Cellos concert on March 29, 2019 would be the last day of my life as I knew it. I'm happy that Scott and I were able to enjoy their music and meet them. Not a bad ending to my life before cancer. The following day would be a defining moment when I felt something "pull" in my back during our run in Hershey. From that day forward, I would continue to adjust to life with cancer.

Today, my primary tumor, in my lower left lobe, is about the size of a pea. This is less than half the size it was when I was first diagnosed. It is being measured in millimeters versus centimeters now. My cancer is stable. I am, however, still considered to be in stage 4, non-small cell lung cancer. Once cancer becomes stage 4 it is systemic, which is a fancy way of saying it is throughout my body. I will always be considered stage 4 even if the cancer is not active. The news on my current health demonstrates that my lung cancer is transitioning from a terminal illness to a chronic disease, similar to diabetes and heart disease. I hope that inspires you! I hope other cancer patients, specifically lung cancer patients, realize how much power they have. This is your life. You and your oncologist make shared decisions on what's best for you.

Now, all that is left for me to do is to continue living with lung cancer. Cancer is part of my life. It doesn't own my mind, body or soul. I believe our lives will return to as close to normal as possible. Perhaps it will never be the same. We know that challenges offer opportunity. Scott and I continue to move forward and live our lives together. We savor each and every moment we have and create many more happy memories. We'll take that sixtieth birthday dream trip someday, though I may be a few years older by then. It will be fun to see how close the real version is to my imagined version. Until then, I'll keep imagining!

Remember the first thing I said when my physician told me that I had a lesion on my spine? My answer is my truth. I said it then, and I'll say it again today with you: "Cancer is not how I'm going to die." I'll continue to move forward and power through whatever lung cancer throws at me. "By hook or by crook," as Dr. Langer would say, "we'll get you there," one day at a time.

Be well, my friends.

Acknowledgments

A special thank you goes to my friend and horn teacher, Jack McCammon. His belief in me made me the horn player I've always hoped to be.

I want to acknowledge the following friends and family for all of their love and support: Corey J. Langer, MD & his wife Mindy, Susie, Dr. Steve & James, Jessica, Caro & Dano, Jack, Susan K, Margaret, Ray, Candy, Merissa, Chris & Antonia, Helena & Marco, Ira & Shirley, Mark & Alison, Dave & Lynn, Cherie, Dean, Eryn, Jacob & Nathan, Alessandra, Alessandro, Alvise, Anna & Angelo, Renato & Paola, Stefania, Lisa, Gary & Jake, Mare & Tom, Melissa & JC, Erica & Chris, Uncle Jimmy, Jimmy Jr. & Michelle, Gus, Maggie & Martina, Andreas & Samia, Candice & Joe, Helen, Grace, Gideon & Shawn, Alisha & Will, Collette, Dusty & Eric, Carolyn G & Dan G, Sean, Benson, James, Pam & Luca, Jen, Yannick & the Philadelphia Orchestra, Andrew & Rupal, Jill, Katie, Joanne, Philippe, Frank, Art, Ken, Panos, Tyron, Stefanie, Julia, Iyla Dominique & Karen, Courtney, Bella, Mike T & Mike M, Darren, Dan & Gladys, Mike H, Kristen, Michael & Sabrina, Cheryl, Joyce, Renee, Delores, Sue, Cassandra, Kooshan, Dr. Linda, Dr. John, Mary E, Jonathan, Lucy & Sam, Jamie, Briana, Rob, Saahil & Nicki, Javier & Elia, Ian & Sarah, Belmary & the Curtis Institute of Music Summerfest staff, Kim & Russ, Reimund & the staff at Gebr. Alexander, Prashant, Filippa, Mike McK, Victoria & Steve, Adriane & Peter, TJ, Maria, Sharon, Kelly, Piero, Amy, Alexa & Melissa, Lauren & Patricia, Gurinder, Ngozi, Carolyn, Mitch, Tom, Mike V, Simson, Dinesh, David S, Sarah, Gordon, Rosemary, Sally, Denise, Scott, Dave &

Laurie, Carey, Cassie, Kyle & Sampty, Babak, Lori, Dan, Bob, Bill, Minnie, Mike F, Jordan, Jessica C, Dr. Linda D, Joe S, Tony, Sarah C, Joanna R, Maria Angela, Debra M, Megan M, Eric M & Sean H, Francis & Eleanor.

Music

THE MUSIC OF LUDWIG VAN BEETHOVEN (1770–1827)

BEETHOVEN, SYMPHONY NO. 1 IN C MAJOR, OP. 21

Sir Georg Solti conducting the Chicago Symphony Orchestra.

(YouTube video, 31:01). Posted by Ahmed Barod on December 4, 2012; accessed by Louis Cesarini February 4, 2021.

https://www.youtube.com/watch?v=Pj2neof3MIs

SYMPHONY NO. 4 IN B♭ MAJOR, OP. 60

Andrés Orozco-Estrada and the Frankfurt Radio Symphony

YouTube video: 36:07. Posted by hr-Sinfonieorchester, March 14, 2016; accessed November 2020.

https://www.youtube.com/watch?v=uGWklkORHJo

SYMPHONIES NO. 5 IN C MINOR, OP. 67 & BEETHOVEN SYMPHONY NO. 6 IN F MAJOR, OP. 68

Yannick Nézet-Séguin & the Philadelphia Orchestra

YouTube video, 1:26:35. Posted by the Philadelphia Orchestra, March 14, 2020; accessed November 2020.

https://www.youtube.com/watch?v=zKWYX5ohadQ

> The program opens with Habibi's "Jeder Baum spricht," followed by Beethoven's 5th and 6th symphonies.

SYMPHONY NO. 5 IN C MINOR, OP. 67

- Minute 10:37 marks the beginning of the first movement.
- Minute 31:27 marks the beginning of the fourth movement.

SYMPHONY NO. 6 IN F MAJOR, OP. 68 "PASTORAL"

- Minute 44:13 marks the beginning of the first movement.
- Minute 1:16:57 marks the beginning of the fifth movement.

SYMPHONY NO. 9 IN D MINOR, OP. 125 "CHORAL"

The Mormon Tabernacle Choir, Eugene Ormandy & the Philadelphia Orchestra

YouTube video, 1:08:14. Posted by soy ink, August 24, 2017; accessed September 2020.

https://www.youtube.com/watch?v=eb_vUFxgtxM

- Minute 15:14 marks the beginning of the second movement.
- Minute 29:06 marks the beginning of the third movement.
- Minute 44:18 marks the opening of the fourth and final movement.

THE MUSIC OF PYOTR ILYICH TCHAIKOVSKY (1840–1893)

THE NUTCRACKER/DE NOTENKRAKER

Yannick Nézet-Séguin & Rotterdams Philharmonisch Orkest

YouTube video, 2:07:01. Posted by NPO Radio 4, January 3, 2011; accessed February 4, 2021 by Louis Cesarini.

https://www.youtube.com/watch?v=tk5Uturacx8

- Minute 29:24 marks when the Christmas Tree begins to grow.
- Minute 35:10 marks the beginning of the Prince leading Clara through the moonlit night pine forest followed by the Waltz of the Flowers.

WESTERN BALLET'S THE NUTCRACKER 2019

YouTube video, 1:36:29. This program was aired on KMVT15 Community Media.

Posted by KMVT December 13, 2019.
Accessed February 4, 2021 by Louis Cesarini.

https://www.youtube.com/watch?v=lYayxixdeUs

- Minute 30:33 marks when the Christmas Tree begins to grow.
- Minute 35:05 marks when the Prince and Clara meet and are escorted through the enchanted forest.

TCHAIKOVSKY SYMPHONY NO. 4 IN F MINOR, OP. 36

Hugo Wolf and the New England Conservatory Philharmonia. Recorded live October 1, 2014 in NEC's Jordan Hall, Boston.

YoouTube video, 44:33. Posted by Ronald van den Berg, February 25, 2015; accessed February 2021.

https://www.youtube.com/watch?v=WsPAXd7VDq8

SYMPHONY NO. 5 IN E MINOR, OP. 64

Eugene Ormandy and the Philadelphia Orchestra, 1974

YouTube video, 48:24. Remastered and posted by Fafner888, August 5, 2016; accessed November 2020.

https://www.youtube.com/watch?v=1_BRAcJmHGA

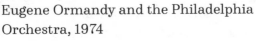

- Minute 15:40 marks the beginning of the second movement. This movement contains the famous French horn solo.

SYMPHONY NO. 6 IN B MINOR, OP. 74 "PATHÉTIQUE"

Eugene Ormandy and the Philadelphia Orchestra

YouTube video, 46:38. Posted by cgoroo, September 30, 2017; accessed September 2020.

https://www.youtube.com/watch?v=mGz8vJeVI8Y

THE MUSIC OF JOHANN SEBASTIAN BACH (1685–1750)

PRELUDE FROM THE PRELUDE AND FUGUE IN C MAJOR, BWV 846 IN THE WELL-TEMPERED CLAVIER: BOOK 1.

Lang Lang, piano

YouTube video, 2:20. Posted by Deutsche Grammophon, June 21, 2019; accessed September 2020.

https://www.youtube.com/watch?v=7ZNXBpO-uEo

LOUIS V. CESARINI: FRENCH HORN

MOZART HORN CONCERTO NO. 3, K 447

Romance (Larghetto) and Allegro. Louis Cesarini's 2018 Curtis Summerfest Audition video YouTube video, 9:07. Posted by Scott Simon, December 2, 2020.

https://www.youtube.com/watch?v=7rmLcf5u_Zw&feature= youtube

BEETHOVEN SEXTET IN E-FLAT MAJOR, OP. 81B FOR TWO HORNS, ADAGIO AND RONDO: ALLEGRO

Curtis Institute of Music Adult Summerfest 2019

Musicians: Michael Smith (piano); Please change to read: Jack McCammon (French horn 1); Louis V. Cesarini (French horn 2)

YouTube video, 11:32. Recorded and posted by Scott Simon, May 19, 2019.

https://youtu.be/MtQTa3OWbt8

BEETHOVEN: SONATA FOR HORN AND PIANO IN F MAJOR, OP. 17

Musicians: Louis V. Cesarini, a.k.a. Louis 2.0 (French horn); Yamaha Disklavier (piano)

YouTube video playlist. Update posted by Louis Cesarini, July 11, 2020.

https://www.youtube.com/playlist?list=PLD3OTBbtv FjmyAorvSgeXVBBIO7gVpVRt

LOUIS & SCOTT: 25ᵀᴴ ANNIVERSARY CELEBRATION

Inglenook winery, Napa Valley, CA, November 2018

Produced by RedSphere Studios, San Francisco, CA (*www.redspherestudios.com*).

https://www.youtube.com/watch?v=gs6lGgQSnHU&t=3s

References and Annotations

NATIONAL COMPREHENSIVE CANCER NETWORK (NCCN)

https://www.nccn.org

....

Guidelines & Clinical Resources

https://www.nccn.org/professionals/physician_gls/default.aspx

FDA-APPROVED INDICATIONS AND PRESCRIBING INFORMATION

Alimta

https://www.alimta.com/hcp/resources?gclid=EAIaIQobCh MItvby-a_c6gIVCZezCh34LgR1EAAYASAAEgKFUPD_BwE

Carboplatin

http://chemocare.com/chemotherapy/drug-info/carboplatin.aspx

Dexamethasone

https://www.webmd.com/drugs/2/drug-1027-5021/ dexamethasone-oral/dexamethasone-oral/details

Doxycycline

https://www.drugs.com/doxycycline.html

Keytruda

https://www.keytruda.com/?src=google&med=cpc&camp=Keytruda+Pan+Tumor+Keytruda+ONLY_Brand_BRND_NA_ENGM_EXCT_TEXT_NA&adgrp=Brand+Keyword_General&kw=keytruda&utm_kxconfid=sq7irm3mh&gclid=EAIaIQobChMI-8S3ga_c6gIVCK_ICh2IvQAMEAAYASAAEgJXpvD_BwE&gclsrc=aw.ds

Lovenox

https://www.drugs.com/lovenox.html

Prednisone

https://www.webmd.com/drugs/2/drug-6007-9383/prednisone-oral/prednisone-oral/details

Tagrisso

https://www.tagrisso.com/stage-4/understanding-lung-cancer/diagnosis.html